FREEDOM FROM ADDICTION

A Hypnotherapist's Guide to Overcoming Addictions and Compulsions

JEREMY WALKER

First published by Jeremy Walker 2018
Copyright © Jeremy Walker
Edited by Shahana Dukhi

All rights reserved. No part of this book may be used or reproduced by any means, graphic, electronic, or mechanical, including photocopying, recording, taping or by any information storage retrieval system without the written permission of the copyright owner except in the case of brief quotations embodied in critical articles and reviews.

Because of the dynamic nature of the Internet, any web addresses or links contained in this book may have changed since publication and may no longer be valid. The views expressed in this work are solely those of the authors and do not necessarily reflect the views of the publisher and the publisher hereby disclaims any responsibility for them.

National Library of Australia
Cataloguing-in-Publication data:
Freedom From Addiction/ Jeremy Walker
ISBN: (sc) 978-0-6484671-0-6
ISBN: (e) 978-0-6484671-1-3

general – nonfiction

Acknowledgements

I want to acknowledge the people who helped make this book possible for you to read.

To my Mum and Al I know I can depend on your love and support with all I endeavour to achieve.

Brad Flynn you gave me the encouragement needed to begin and persevere with this project. Thank you.

Jarrod L'Estrange I appreciate your continued support for my work. You help me impact more lives with my message.

Karen Mc Dermott for helping me navigate the publishing process. Thank you.

Thank you to my teachers in Hypnotherapy, Addiction Treatment, The Demartini Method and Psychosomatic Therapy. Your wisdom, love and knowledge impact me to this day.

Thank you to the clients who entrust their care to me. Your courage to rise above the toughest challenges inspires.

My fiancé and Editor Shahana Dukhi. You have been by my side the entire time writing. You helped me create the best book I can. Your diligence to produce excellent work is second to none.

CONTENTS

Introduction	1
Difficulties in Breaking Addictions	6
My Story: Misadventures on Drugs	15
The Subconscious Mind	30
Dealing with Stress	38
Parent Goals	51
The Easy Way to Be Disciplined	57
Food: The Most Complicated Addiction	64
False Cravings	86
My Journey to Mastery	95
Pain and Drugs	99
Identity: Who You Are	110
Environment	120
Addictions as False Security	126
List of 50 Reasons People Have Compulsions and Addictions	133
Addictions Create What You Don't Want	135
Revealing What You Need	142
Walker Addictions Removal Process (WARP)	148
Conclusion	161

*The best way to predict your future,
is to create it.*

Introduction

I am writing this book as if we are talking with each other face to face. Feel free to receive it in this way. My intention for writing, is to help you be free from your persistent compulsion or addiction. I will show you a path forward, if you have a behaviour you would like to transform.

From the outset, I'm not here to judge your addiction or compulsion, there is enough of that already. In fact, judgement can often reinforce an addiction. People on the outside seem to be taking something away from you, while the addiction seems like the answer.

I have always been interested in addictions and compulsions. It's intrigued me how a person DOES something that they DON'T want to. Is it due to a lack of impulse control? Is it related to self-worth? Is it a force of habit? Does addiction become part of identity? We'll explore all of these fascinating questions together.

Why would you want to be free from addiction? Perhaps your addiction is causing major problems. Your compulsions are impacting your work and finances. It is costing you physically and mentally. It is straining the relationships with people you care about.

I've heard clients say many times, "I don't know why I have an addiction. I want to change, but I just go back to it again and again. I feel anxious, like I'm missing something without it." The addiction might make them feel in control temporarily, but really they are out of control.

I remember playing poker machines in my early 20s and money would start to run out. I told myself I would have enough for a good time with friends and get a cab home. That's not what happened though.

I had awareness that I was going to lose, but it's like there was a force, that compelled me to keep playing right down to the last spin, as if on auto pilot. A short time later, I had no money to re-join friends or get a cab. I'd walk home, feeling empty and embarrassed. This experience of **creating the results we don't want in life**, is what we'll call an inner conflict.

Your compulsion or addiction might be losing $100 to a poker machine each week, burying yourself in debt buying shoes, eating that chocolate dessert every night (even though you said you wouldn't), to secretly drinking through the day to 'function' at work.

There's a part of you that wants to be free from the addiction, however there is a part of you that also wants to keep it. At a fundamental level, there are benefits to stopping the behaviour as well as benefits you get by continuing the behaviour. We are going to place a spotlight on what you get from addiction, so you can see a clearer path to be free from it.

At different times in this book, I'll invite you to turn to page 158. Here you can fill in a table, which will give you insights about your compulsion or addiction. We'll discuss various ideas, then bring them all together with the **Walker Addiction Removal Process**.

I have put together 4 example addictions, so you can see a path to move forward for each one. There are 2 blank tables you can use for any compulsion or addiction you want to work on. Each chapter will reveal context and deeper meaning to the **WARP**, used to break addictions.

I will share cases from my clinic showing how transformations take place in a session. All names have been changed to protect people's identity. The stories are accurate, taking into account that small details change with memory. The integrity of the stories are intact.

Many, I work with feel embarrassed and guilty about their addiction. These emotions can blind us in looking for the positive intention behind our behaviour. This is the first idea I will invite you to explore.

Addictions have a positive intention behind them. Rather than judgement, ask, what do I get from that?

I'll often ask clients what they get out of smoking cigarettes, overeating, or drinking alcohol. Most say, "Nothing, it's bad," but within a few minutes we get somewhere between 6-12 different reasons, why they do what they do.

A gentleman I worked with on alcohol reduction had 25 positive things he got out of drinking. Rather than focusing on drinking being bad, we focused on finding alternatives to satisfy what he gets from alcohol. We worked on each component of his drinking habit.

A craving has a need behind it that can be difficult to pinpoint. I have observed in many cases, when habits are substituted correctly, cravings can disappear, or become much more manageable.

You will have a vastly expanded view of addiction by completing the exercises in this book. Once you've done it, you'll be able to apply this learning to any compulsion or addiction you have. You'll be able to see why you do what you do and able to see it in others as well.

Questioning everything is far better than having the perfect answer. Take special notice of something that inspires or challenges you, both will give access to transformation. Write down and explore in the real world any idea that grabs your attention.

The goal of any addiction work, should be to reach the point, where you don't have to use willpower any more to fight it. In my opinion, if you're still craving the old behaviour, you haven't received full service. Therapy is complete, when you no longer have inner conflict.

There is a difference between resisting addiction and being free from it.

Again I'm not saying any particular behaviour is bad; smoking a joint, shopping for your favourite shoes, or eating ice-cream, only you'd want to be in control of that behaviour. We will look at compulsions and addictions in great detail, from my personal experiences and conducting thousands of sessions. We will explore what has worked to be free from addiction.

Difficulties in Breaking Addictions

Whilst assisting in transforming an addiction, one of the first steps I'll take, is to find out why they do what they do. Uncovering this lets me know a number of things. Does the person have awareness of why they have an addiction? Are the reasons simply boredom or something deeper, like trying to escape pain?

Compulsions and addictions are present in your life for a reason. Internal motivators to resist change can be strong and there is a fear of giving it up. Knowing your motivators, gives you power, to move forward.

What people get at a deeper level from their compulsion or addiction, can vastly vary. Rather than pointing out to someone their addiction is bad, you can ask, "What needs and wants is it satisfying? What purpose is that serving for you?" The answers to those questions, might surprise you.

Case Study Jeff

Jeff was the state manager of a sales company in Queensland. He had a girlfriend, a high income and trained hard in martial arts. He came to see me to reduce his alcohol consumption, which on some days would be 12-16 drinks. He didn't drink every day but when he did, it was a lot.

When I work with someone, I expect they will have a breakthrough (large or small) in every session. In my Alcohol Reduction Program I suggested that he have alcohol free days and set a 'healthy drinking limit.' An agreement was made that 4 units was an absolute maximum limit to set.

After his first appointment he had kept to his maximum limit of 4, on all but one occasion. He was half way through his 5th drink at a party and vomited. This shocked him, because he used to be able to stomach more than 12. The hypnosis had worked and his body now had a strong deterrent against passing 4 drinks.

Important note: I hadn't suggested he would vomit, if he exceeded his limit. This automatic reaction came from his body's new truth, that he was a healthy drinker, who could only have a maximum of 4 drinks on any given day. Having 5 drinks violated this truth and his subconscious mind found a way to correct it.

Jeff and I explored his relationship with alcohol a little deeper. We looked for what he enjoyed about drinking. To our surprise, he listed 25 things he got from drinking alcohol. These included; having fun, lowering inhibitions, being the life of the party, to stop overthinking and enhanced sexual performance.

Who would I be to take that list away from him? I didn't!

What we did was work on a plan to meet all of his needs and wants from equal or even better sources than alcohol. Through diligent work, he found at least 5 ways to satisfy every single one of the things he was getting from alcohol, from other sources.

Jeff discovered the positive intention behind his drinking and opened himself to looking for alternatives. Because all of his reasons for drinking are being satisfied, he drinks much less. Jeff still chooses to drink on occasion. He does it purposely now and is progressing well with his martial arts training.

If Jeff had quit drinking because 'it was bad,' he would have got back on it harder when under pressure in the future. Why? Because he would not have created new ways to meet his needs and wants. Judgements keep people stuck. What you resist, persists (until you find a balanced perspective).

Because Jeff is getting what he needs, the change is long lasting. This is the power of uncovering the 'motivators' for why we do what we do. Jeff has alternatives that are equal to or better than drinking alcohol. His energy is up, he is fitter and his mood is improved. He will likely not go back to the pattern of binge drinking.

If you try to quit something because you feel guilt and shame about it, you are in a position of dis-empowerment. You will try to quit because you think 'it's bad' and anger when you start again. Continue to explore in your life what you are getting from your habits.

There is a solution for every person and I have not met anyone who can't stop their addiction, with some perseverance. There is a **need** and **alternative** not yet revealed to them. For some it will be enough to discover the purpose of their addiction. For others, due to circumstances in life, it will take much more work.

Imagine trying to quit a long term habit, without knowing the truth about why you do it. Society blinds us into thinking we are doing something bad. That is dis-empowerment training. Shame, shame, shame. It's pretty hard to support ourselves physically and mentally when we don't even know what we need thus addiction continues!

At this point I'll invite you to view pages 133 and 134. This is a list of 50 reasons people have compulsions and addictions. Consider which of these drive the behaviour you have. You can use your top 5 reasons in the **WARP**.

Case Study Nadia

In 2016, Nadia had visited me to significantly reduce sugar intake, which had become a compulsive habit for her. During her second appointment she stated that she wanted to give up sugar, in all forms, forever!

She wanted this to include chocolate, lollies, sauces, yoghurt and fruit (which all have sugar in some form). Imagine trying to manage this level of restriction. It is not realistic and somewhere in the back of her mind, she would have known this too.

The all or nothing approach with food habits often does more damage than good. I offer the distinction between a **short term restrictive diet** and a plan for **lifelong health and energy**. You may have experienced losing 15kg on a restrictive diet before, but what happens after you stop the diet?

The short term strategy is repressing something 'bad' which causes the behaviour to bounce back with a vengeance. You've tried that before and know it does not work. The longer term strategy asks, "What does your body and mind need to be healthy AND energised, which also is practical?"

Back to Nadia. I took her through the **WARP**, to find the internal motivators that led her to overeating of sugar. At first she was very resistant to the idea of the sugar having benefits, asserting, "Sugar is bad, I don't get anything from it!!" This is one of only a few times someone has yelled at me in an appointment.

Despite this, within 20 minutes we had 13 reasons and positive emotional attachments that relate to her eating sugar. One of them was that a certain type of chocolate reminded her of her Mother's love, who lived in another country. She was eating to fill a void of loneliness, which made her feel closer to family.

Remember, if we do not get something from our compulsions and addictions, we wouldn't do them.

Chocolate or any other food, is not bad or good. You'd want to note the results it is producing in your life. In Nadia's case sugar was leading to weight gain she was uncomfortable with and was consuming her mind.

We explored alternative ways to meet the needs of her 13 reasons, including numerous ways she can feel love from Mum. These new alternatives included genuine connection with her Mum via phone, planning holidays to go home and more connection with family here in Australia.

The sugar was a poor substitute for love. Nadia felt shame about her compulsion to eat chocolate. Shame is rarely a catalyst for positive change as it is such a heavy emotion. It tends to keep people stuck and retreating in safety on the inside which eventually leads to lashing out, or pretending the problem doesn't exist, in order to avoid facing it.

Shame is a false belief that part of yourself is wrong. Shame is letting you know there is a part of yourself that needs **love and self-acceptance.** I won't pretend it's different to this. If you don't clear out guilt and shame, it will continue to run your mind.

Many people living with shame wish it would just go away but have no idea why it's there. Shame is a signal from your mind that you believe falsely that some part of you is invalid or bad.

Can you look closely at yourself and ask, "Is this self-judgement actually true, at all?" "Who said so?" You will find all negative judgement to be false, when you look closely at it. **Judgement is a comparison as to how you think you should be rather than accepting who you are.**

Self-enquiry, shadow work and self-acceptance is your path here. Join me in my Self Mastery and Transformation study group online for more on this and other topics.

https://facebook.com/groups/selfmasteryandtransformation

It is possible through self-enquiry to transform shame into gratitude. Take the part of you, you believe is wrong and look for the positive reason it is there. It could be a strategy for protection, to gain something, appear acceptable to others, to avoid responsibility or many other possible things. Every part of you is okay and has a purpose.

Nadia had become angry at one point in our work together, yelling loudly in my office. She was still holding on to the belief that sugar was bad, despite revealing 13 benefits of it being in her life. There was guilt and shame that was blocking her from making a full breakthrough.

Earlier in our work together, I hadn't realised the depth of judgement she was experiencing around sugar. The path forward for Nadia would involve processing the guilt and shame she feels. I was introducing the possibility that she is whole and complete. She was fighting for the limitation that she and sugar are bad.

No one ever got better by believing part of them was wrong.

The reason I challenged her belief that sugar was bad, is because that was the same old belief she was carrying for 20 years. It never once empowered her to transform. If you carry the same beliefs about your addiction and yourself, you won't get different results in the future.

Sugar may well be bad, but if we weren't getting something from it we wouldn't do it. We focus on what it is you get from addiction and that shows you what you need in life. By finding the reasons we do what we do, we clear out a lot of guilt and shame. Over time we see that we weren't bad but doing the best we could with the options available.

Clearing out these types of heavy emotions means we end up making better decisions. Many eat more when they feel ashamed, to comfort themselves. So, the shame about eating sugar, can contribute to eating sugar! We may all be looking for comfort and love, so we'll explore multiple ways we can get those needs fulfilled in this book.

My Story: Misadventures on Drugs

In writing this book, I thought about times I have had a compulsive behaviour run my mind. I've had a dozen different compulsive behaviours in my life, all of which were damaging in some way. These were as simple as being hooked on video games for hours on end, eating sugar even though it was continuing to inflame my chronic fatigue, to a regular marijuana and drug habit.

As a growing teenager alcohol and marijuana were easy to come by. We stood in awe as one of the kids down the street showed us his Dad's shed where $40,000 of marijuana achingly bulged in large plastic bags. He would grab handfuls and sell it to us for a fraction of what it was really worth.

Another place we easily acquired drugs was at a friend's house where Steven had been smoking since he was 6 years old and his brother, 5. They lived with their parents into their early 20s and lived to smoke every day.

We would basically hang out, muck around and play video games. I remember the very first time I smoked weed over there, I took a big toke and immediately passed out. I wasn't used to smoking marijuana along with cigarette tobacco and the weed was very strong.

My best drug taking friend and I broke into the local surf club one night. There was a piece of wood holding the door shut, so we wedged a stick under the door and leveraged it, until the wood came out. We wanted to watch TV in there and smoke weed and had no malicious intent except for use of the place to hang out and get high.

We hadn't counted on one of the locals nearby spying a light on in the club and calling the police. We had no time to escape as we heard them coming up the stairs. Our push bikes, bong and backpacks were in plain sight, when they walked in. We quickly ducked further into the building down another set of stairs to hide.

I positioned myself behind the rescue boat and my friend was hiding in a cupboard. We were both found in under 2 minutes. Thankfully in the state of New South Wales there were new laws offering multiple cautions for kids involved in drugs. On different occasions I was cautioned twice for possessing drugs and once for driving on a golf course in my van.

What this meant early on in my life was, I hadn't suffered any serious consequences from taking drugs although I did feel horrible for Mum who was crying when she had to pick me up from the police station. Aside from that, the arrests made me more aware of avoiding police but didn't stop me from taking drugs for very long.

Unrestricted by life or authority figures, at 16 years old I basically did whatever I wanted. At times I had the afternoon off from school and together with a friend we would drink, smoke and swim in the ocean. I did what I wanted and adjusted strategy if I was raising too much suspicion.

I failed spectacularly at avoiding suspicion one day at school. On this particular day, I went home for lunch and smoked weed before going back for afternoon classes. In class, my face started to turn green. I then put my arms out on the desk in front of me and went to sleep. This is often called 'greening out.'

After about 40 minutes, the school bell rang and I opened my eyes to see our teacher shaking his head at me. He knew! As I lifted my head to get up, dozens of staples and rolled up pieces of paper fell out of my hair. Classmates had put them there while I was asleep, the teacher must have seen, but let them do it.

I used drugs regularly from the ages of 14 to 23 and was an experimental drug taker starting with cigarettes, alcohol and marijuana as many do. Once I'd turned 18, I began using ecstasy and speed with the added option of going down the herbal path, trying hallucinogens, seeds and liquid stimulants.

One week I would have some herbal highs and just enjoy good vibes. Another week I might smoke marijuana or take ecstasy and liking the experience of a variety of different sensations, careful not to become dependent on any one drug in particular.

I had convinced myself it was okay to take all these drugs, as long I didn't do it too often and no 'one drug' controlled my life. All up I have taken 19 different legal and illegal drugs. Every action we take has consequences. I was yet to experience mine, so I went on my merry way. Of course, a crash was coming.

Reckless with my job and myself, as a kid, I had crashed my pushbike a few times, lucky to avoid injury. As a young adult I sometimes was under the influence of marijuana at work, drank alcohol and drove and was highly irresponsible in general.

My Van, Marijuana and a Tree

On a hapless night at about 11:00pm, I was having a great time driving in heavy rain stoned on marijuana when my van slid into a suburban garden. I was stuck in the middle of 3 large bushes. I couldn't move the van forwards at all, but managed to reverse out. In doing so I uprooted one of the trees, which was now stuck underneath. The bush was about 3 feet long.

My plan from then on was to drive to a local park, to see if I could pull it out. I was so high that I drove into a retirement home instead. The dragging of that bush underneath the van was extremely loud in the still of the night and started smoking as it dragged along the bitumen.

I must have woken half the retirement home with the noise of the scraping tree and reversing in and out of several driveways. I was lost. What is easy when you are straight can be incredibly difficult when you are stoned. I knew if I didn't get out of there soon, the police would be called and I would be up for a police conviction this time. I was starting to panic.

Disorientated in the middle of this retirement home having no idea in which direction I was facing. I said to myself, "just keep turning left and you'll get out." I don't know how, but I did make it out before I got caught doing something ridiculous again.

I phoned my cousin that lived nearby who said yes to my request of hiding my van at his place until morning. I stayed over at his house and was relieved the ordeal was all over. My old brown van and adopted tree, all tucked away safely in his garage.

About a week later I went back to inspect damage to the garden I drove into. Yeah it didn't look pretty. Thankfully those bushes were the only things that got hurt and I hadn't killed or injured myself or anyone else with all the reckless stuff I had been doing.

From time to time in my drug taking days, I would stop using everything for 3 months which was a control measure I had in place to make sure I was in charge of my mind, I've always had a high price on it. Because of this I wouldn't say I was an addict, but I definitely had a drug problem and compulsive habits.

During my drug taking days, I conducted research for all the information on different drugs and plants wanting to know the upsides and risks of everything I took. Government sites, books written by addicts, articles by herbalists and online forums, where drug users would post their personal experiences online sufficed.

Did you know for example, marijuana isn't the only plant you can smoke? There are actually several hundred different ones you could try for relaxation or a mild high. Many have no psycho-active properties at all which means they don't cause hallucinations.

I'm not talking about synthetic weed but organic plants that are legal with some even possessing health benefits. As part of experimenting, I explored this world of plants and legal highs and manned a market stall to sell them in Northern NSW.

I was selling everything from Cats Claw (Uncaria tormentosa), which is known as an anti-cancer herb, to liquid stimulants made from legal and illegal ingredients. I realised as time went on that people were more interested in the 'semi-legal drugs' and less in medicine.

I started to feel like I was becoming a drug dealer. This didn't fit in with why I had started the market stall in the first place. I wanted to help and educate people and after nearly 2 years I left it all behind... I was still using drugs at this time but didn't want to sell them.

I loved the way drugs made me feel. I'd be high, get tingles in my body, have increased sexual performance, see beautiful hallucinations and experience soaring bouts of confidence which led to my connecting with people.

From Drug Use to Hypnotherapist

From 2006 onwards, consequences of drug use were catching up with me. I experienced a slow deterioration in physical health. It happened in a way where I didn't notice at first. One day I woke up sore, tired, with an aching body and realised I'd been feeling this way for months on end. My sex drive having gone way down, I just didn't feeling like it unless I was on something.

My Story: Misadventures on Drugs

It was around a year later that I experienced serious digestion problems, anxiety and chronic fatigue. Chronic fatigue takes shape in 1 of 2 ways. It either happens very quickly, or creeps in and you don't quite notice it at first. Mine happened slowly and begun several months after stopping regular drug use.

I worked out the contributors to my chronic fatigue were; high physical stress, poor diet and drug use which led to digestion problems. I ended up dropping in weight from 68kg down to 60kg. I swore I wouldn't allow myself to go below 60kg (about 132lbs in weight).

Daily life was tough. Digestion was of such poor quality at the time that I would eat a small breakfast at 6:00am, leave for work, be home at 9:00am and feel undigested food still there in my stomach and on those days I would lay down and take a nap. My body was spent.

It was at this time that I had commenced my spiritual and healing journey and over the next several years, I dedicated myself to restoring my body, energy levels and mind. By restoring my gut health with clean eating and attending hundreds of tai chi classes the chronic fatigue eventually did heal.

Across the world there are people who want to change but aren't able to find what helps bring about real transformation! Some aren't exactly sure what health advice to follow and this is what I became engrossed in. Health is by no means defined only by the weight we are, it comes about by **truly supporting ourselves mentally and physically**.

Post drugs I read abundantly, consuming 2-3 books a week on health, human behaviour and how to transform addictions. I moved to Brisbane QLD, in 2009 and began studying formally in Psychosomatic Therapy, Hypnotherapy, NLP and The Demartini Method.

I have been blessed to learn from some of the world's masters in Mind/Body Health and Transformational Therapies. I discovered that with correct systems in place, change was possible for me and others. In recovering the relationship with self, physical as well as mental energy substantially increased.

I apply the above transformational therapies to help 'get results.' This might sound obvious but there exists types of therapy work that are just for venting and support. My work is to help people master their thoughts, emotions, compulsions and addictions, so no negative pattern can run their life again.

I work with people locally in Brisbane and by phone worldwide to overcome their compulsions and addictions. Many I see in sessions are; nurses, teachers, managers, miners, busy mums, hardworking dads, famous actors and business owners. All are different people with one commonality, they have a compulsive behaviour they want to control.

Many have had their compulsion or addiction for up to 30 or 40 years. They have usually controlled it before, for a short time but seem to go back to their 'old ways' when faced with the pressures of life. This includes those who have been on 10+ diets and the weight returns, cigarette smokers, people who gamble and alcohol abusers to name a few.

I used drugs for the pleasure and highs. I consider myself very fortunate in that I hadn't used drugs to avoid pain or in avoidance of dealing with issues. When it comes to displaying any compulsion or addiction, you are likely to fall into one or both of these categories.

1) You have an addiction to avoid or get away from something negative.
2) You have an addiction to experience or gain something positive.

My hook on drugs was not to escape pain, as it is for some. Intuitively, from an early age I knew, "Don't take anything if I am in a negative head-space." This is an important safe-guard to help protect your mental health, if you have stuff going on for you right now.

I found my Dad dead at 16 years old, after the funeral everyone was having beers and I thought, "Isn't this the sort of time I should be clear of intoxicants?" It's been my experience of not having seen anyone cope with life better by getting drunk or taking drugs, quite the contrary really.

I knew there would be difficult emotions, I also believed these types of incidents would shape how I deal with grief in the future. Drinking is one option and allowing grief to process naturally is another (accepting having to deal with a wide range of feelings, without trying to change them).

Children and Drugs

Children are introduced to drugs from age 12 or younger. It will likely happen at school or at a friend's house. You don't want their first knowledge about drugs to come from another child or worse, someone older trying to take advantage.

It can be scary broaching this topic with your child, we fear that talking about drugs will somehow encourage them to seek it. As a parent you are in the best position to help kids understand the risks and reasons people partake of drugs.

"Children who have benefited from an open, trusting channel of communication about difficult issues in early years carry that protection into their teenage years and

are more likely to make wise decisions." Lois Sailsbury – President of Children Now

The issue of drugs could be addressed as early as 8 or 10 years old. Make these conversations as natural as you can by finding 'teaching moments.' A report on the nightly news, a smoker outside the supermarket or a story on social media can provide an opportunity to engage.

Chatting to your kids before one of their friend's at school does, is the goal here. You have a better chance of keeping them safe by educating them about the risk and reality of drugs (age appropriate). With education children can feel confident turning down an offer of drugs.

We tell kids, "drugs are bad and they'll ruin your life." The problem this presents is a closing off of communication in maintaining too strong a position against drugs. Children by nature are intensely curious. If you tell your preteen that all drugs are bad, they will smell bullshit and try them anyway, just like you did, to find the truth.

Give children excessive education, not excessive threats.

The more educated children are, the more empowered they are to make informed decisions. You could say something like this to your teen, or preteen:

"Taking drugs once probably won't kill you, but it is more likely that it will lead to an encounter with the police, getting into a fight, crashing a car, becoming sick or falling pregnant. These are real life consequences!

Children use drugs for a variety of reasons, giving in to pressure from friends and others yet may use to escape pain. It remains a very temporary experience that can have dire long-term effects. Drugs will ultimately cause the opposite of what you want.

There are some who smoke cigarettes to be cool but take a closer look at smokers, they don't actually look cool at all do they? People drink alcohol to have fun but hangovers and vomiting are also a reality of drinking. It looks fun and cool, but it's dirty and painful as well."

Give your child a chance to respond. Conduct an initial conversation without an interrogative tone and steer clear from demanding that they are to never use drugs. If the conversation progresses on to where they reveal that one of the kids at school smokes pot at home or someone had white powder in their school bag, you now have an opportunity to provide them with guidance.

Try to not be angry that they are only telling you about it at this point. You might praise them for engaging in the talk. At this time you can encourage them not to mind anyone else's drugs if they get asked to and assure that they can come to you to ask any questions.

Although your teen may not give you the benefit of a big thank you for educating them on drugs, they will however remember at least some of what you tell them. I remembered something my Dad had told me 10 years after he'd said it. Maybe I was slow in getting it or it just made more sense at a later stage in life.

Setting up support structures to keep your kids safe is also wise. These suggestions may be valuable:

- "Call us if your friend is drink driving. We will come and pick you up immediately at any time."
- "Don't take anything if you're unsure as to where it came from. Only accept unopened drinks."
- Set up activities for your kids with their friends that are highly enjoyable, fun, active and also healthy.
- Keep an eye on their mental health in general.
- Get them involved in sport, dancing, martial arts, community or other activities.
- Get your teenager setting goals (Goals revolving around education, career, money, health, relationships).

- Encourage time spent with older role models of the same sex.

The Subconscious Mind

I want to make a distinction between your conscious and subconscious mind, to form a foundation for the chapters ahead. For the sake of simplicity, let's say a 'subconscious mind' handles things which are outside your awareness and a 'conscious mind' is the part used for making new choices.

Traits of a Conscious Mind:

- Logical and rational.
- Makes new choices.
- Uses willpower.
- Has limited problem solving ability.

Traits of a Subconscious Mind:

- Where thoughts and emotions originate.
- Controls bodily functions like blinking and breathing.
- Has unlimited problem solving ability.
- Holds on to habits and patterns of behaviour.

You can choose to control blinking if you want to but only for a short time. A few minutes on and you'll forget about it, your subconscious mind will again take over that role, keeping your eyes moist and protected.

Trying to quit an addiction is like this for most. You battle with willpower to control something that has become an automatic response. As time goes on you lose focus and revert to hair twirling, craving sex, taking drugs, or smoking a cigarette.

The craving to repeat behaviour over and over again, comes from the subconscious mind. This means you will have trouble in simply willing urges and cravings to go away. No one ever 'chooses' to be addicted. There are wants and needs the addiction is attempting to satisfy outside your awareness.

Transformation happens when the conscious and subconscious mind want the same thing, at the same time. At a deeper level, you want something else, more than the urge to repeat an old behaviour or the impulse is simply no longer.

Hypnotherapy

Hypno-therapy is an effective treatment that works with the subconscious mind. In a relaxed state of hypnosis, conscious thoughts slow down and we can communicate directly with the subconscious.

The Subconscious Mind

In a state of hypnosis you are relaxed yet aware of what is going on around you. A similar state to when half-awake in the morning. You can vaguely hear noises around you, but are not really thinking yet.

A part of the mind which engages in analysing slows down in hypnosis and one can accept new possibilities, often times using no willpower at all. The ultimate goal of hypnosis is to help make a change without having to battle yourself in achieving it.

One reason why hypnotherapy is so effective for transformation, is that it changes your response to difficult situations in hours versus months or years. With your subconscious mind free of inner conflict the need for willpower is not needed to break addiction.

Remember, you want to work at a subconscious level where your problem would have started. Thoughts, emotions, compulsions and addictions are all governed by your subconscious mind. During times of treating clients with hypnotherapy I have witnessed interesting transformations.

A gentleman I worked with smoked 60 cigarettes and drank 20 cups of coffee daily. This gentleman did quit smoking though interestingly, his coffee intake went from 20 down to 4 per day without even thinking about it. "It just happened," he said.

During thousands of hypnosis sessions which I've facilitated in people come out of an hour session and report feeling free and having the ability to breathe deeply once more. Is the subconscious mind capable of quitting 40 year addictions in an hour? Does the belief in our own inner power make the difference?

I Sent You Two Boats and a Helicopter

This is the story of a man who was trapped on the roof of his house, during a flood. It rained and rained for hours. The man in his living room quickly realised he would have no escape from floodwaters that had surrounded the house. The man climbed up on to the roof and knew that he would be okay. He was a firm believer in God. His God would protect him.

It kept raining and the water had reached the roof of his house and nearly reached his ankles. A little while later a boat came by and the guy in it said, "jump in quick, I'll save you. I will take you with us." "No thanks," said the man. "I'm a firm believer in God. He will rescue me." The boat drove away.

It kept raining and water had reached his waist now. Another boat came by and the guy in the boat said: "You look like you need some help. Jump in before it's too late." "No," said the man. "I'm a firm believer in God. He will rescue me. I'm waiting for God."

It still rained and the water reached his neck. Miraculously a helicopter came by and a rope was thrown down. The rescuer in the helicopter yelled, "Grab the rope quick, we're here to save you my friend. "No," yelled the man, through the pouring rain. "I'm a firm believer in God. He will rescue me. I know he will."

The helicopter crew begged the man to take this lifeline, but the man was firm in his belief. He was waiting. Eventually the helicopter flew away. It kept on raining and the man drowned.

When the man died, he went to Heaven. When entering Heaven, he had an interview with God. After a polite greeting and sitting down, the man demanded, "Where the hell were you? I waited and waited. I was sure you would rescue me, as I have been a firm believer in you all my life and have only done well by others. So where were YOU when I needed you?"

God stared blankly at the man. He had seen this before, but it still surprised even the All Mighty. God scratched his head and answered: "I sent you a rescue boat and you turned it away. I sent you a second rescue boat and you turned it away. I sent you a rescue helicopter and you turned it away too, what the hell were YOU waiting for?"

In life, I tend to follow this philosophy: Have faith like there is a God, and work hard like there isn't one. I believe that everything is as an Act of God working in my favour. When life appears to not work in my favour I look for a learning, meaning and gratitude for what is… What *you* need may be in front of you right now and you are missing it.

Directing Your Subconscious Mind

An impulse to act on a behaviour, comes from your subconscious mind. You may have never decided to create an addiction to drugs or any other addiction for that matter. The original decision took place behind the scenes without your knowledge, by your subconscious.

You want to work with the subconscious part of the mind, when changing any compulsion or addiction. Just as you can't will anger to go away when you are in the middle of it, you cannot simply will your addiction to go away without deeper work on yourself. There are steps to take when breaking addictions that work 'behind the scenes.' These help support you physically and mentally to do it.

Think of it as if it were a theatre show. The audience sees actors performing a successful piece of work that lasts for an hour. What the audience doesn't see is the teamwork it took to make it happen, the actors investing months of practice and the director, who influenced every movement on stage.

The actors are the conscious mind, they are the result of repetitive training. The more they practise what they do, the better they get. The director is the one behind the scenes that brings complex ideas together. The director is like your subconscious mind.

The theatre show will only be as good the director makes it. Your life will only be as good as the culmination of habits that originate from your subconscious mind. If you are creating a show with no director, you have a group of actors without clear guidance.

To take the metaphor to its point of relevance for you... If the director is directing the actors, then who is directing the director? Many of the strategies in this book are designed to work with your subconscious mind, so you can train to not just work with willpower but to enrol your deeper power, via your subconscious mind. You can *direct* your director.

Traditional coaching will have you get out of your comfort zone and use will-power but you already know this only works for a short time. You want to train your mind to see your addiction differently and to take new action to override old patterns.

The **WARP** will use a special series of questions to get your mind working on your side. The subconscious believes it benefits from your addiction. To overcome a behaviour pattern you want to satisfy the needs and wants your subconscious is getting from the addiction.

Dealing with Stress

An important step on your freedom from addiction journey is to manage your stress better. I have observed that people with high levels of mental stress find it harder to break an addiction as compared to one who stresses lesser. Not impossible, just harder.

This person is more likely to skip breakfast and have a diet of quick, processed foods. They are more likely to work long hours or do shift work and likely to have strained relationships with family. Many people I see in sessions use their compulsion or addiction as a release from stress in their life.

When a person's primary method in dealing with difficult emotions is unhealthy, it can create a dependence on that behaviour. You don't want to become dependent on something unhealthy to change how you feel. If you have a cigarette, overeat or drink alcohol every time that you are stressed, you aren't dealing with the reasons the stress is there.

What do you do when you experience stress? Do you work on solving the problem that has caused stress, or pretend it's not there? Do you share your emotions with others, or shut down? Be aware of what you do when stress comes up.

It is likely you have drank alcohol, eaten chocolate or smoked a cigarette at the end of a long day, at least once before in your life. 99 people out of 100 would have. There is no problem in doing that as long as that is not an **only** or **primary** way to deal with stress.

I'll often ask clients, "What do you do when you have a bad day? What helps you release stress that is also healthy?" Many reply with, "Nothing" or "I don't have the time." We work on expanding their options in responding to stress, to find things that will work for them.

If a primary way of dealing with stress is avoidance, this will cause problems for you in the long run. It is possible to approach stress in a way that is powerful and healthy.

Taking Responsibility

Case Study Josh

In late 2017 I worked with a gentleman named Josh. He was a guy in his mid-thirties who worked in the Pilbara Region in Western Australia. This is a remote area known for mining that employs thousands of fly-in, fly-out workers.

Josh told me early in our time working together he was the sort of guy that didn't take responsibility for anything in life. He would just let issues slide until things became too difficult to bear. Easier to avoid things and deal with it all later, he thought. He was letting himself down in the areas of health, relationships and wealth. Dealing with it later, wasn't working. Rather than shame him about his past choices or encourage him to be more responsible in the future, I asked him how his stress levels were. He answered that "they were through the roof." Already I had a hint of this because I knew he was not solving any of his problems.

Stress relief is found by solving problems.

We discussed his goals and stress reduction. He had the realisation that pretending his problems weren't there, had led to his mental overwhelm. I asked him to visualise what his life would be like if every one of his stresses was resolved. "What would it be like if every single thing in your life was complete and you get to finally experience peace?"

I then observed relief start to spread over his face and body as if washing away years of unresolved stresses. When we acknowledge stress, work on a plan to reduce it and take action, there is no stress.

Keep in mind here, that the stress you experience is doing its job. It is simply making you aware that you have unresolved problems that need your attention. You need a good plan to deal with it, one that genuinely works.

Once Josh placed **attention** on his thoughts and genuinely **decided** to work through the problems he had, the stress started to go away. When the plan is good enough, stress doesn't need to be there. Literally.

Stress is a message that your strategy for dealing with problems needs adjusting.

I have never met anyone who wants to have less health, love and money but some people get stuck in a cycle of choosing destruction over creating what they want in life... It takes a similar amount of energy to solve your stresses, as it does to be overwhelmed, by ignoring them. We might as well get to work on solving problems because we know avoiding them doesn't work.

3 Approaches You Can Take To Deal with Stress

Have you ever witnessed a family member or friend who seems really stressed out and you ask, "Why don't you just relax?" That question has never worked because they have not changed the conditions that have caused the stress. We would not have stress if we didn't think something was 'wrong,' therefore stress reduction must, address the thing we perceive as wrong.

When in the middle of an overwhelming stressful experience, it's pretty hard to see anything but the stress. What we can do, is break down the issue into smaller parts (like we will do with your addiction by the end of this book). You can make stress easier to manage, by working on smaller parts that make up your particular problem.

You can view stressful thoughts and emotions as a signal that 1 of these 3 things are needed. Consider 1 or all of the following ways to approach stress. Determine which ones best fit your situation.

1) Action is needed to correct something in your life.
2) There is something to let go of.
3) A change is needed in your psychology.

1. Resolve the Cause of Your Stress

This method works to reduce stress by solving whatever is causing the problem you are stressed about. In early 2017 I had a financial related stress. I saw that I was going to be $10,000 short on cash for the next 4-5 months which meant expenses I was going to be unable to pay for.

For several weeks I worried about being short of cash. "Would everything I've worked for vanish? Would things ever improve? What was I to do?" One day I dedicated some time to working out how I could make up the shortfall of cash. Within 1 hour, I'd made up 80% of the money with a new business plan and a few other ideas.

This taught me a valuable lesson about stress. For weeks I wasn't even working on my finances, when I created a plan to deal with it, the stress immediately left me! When a problem causing the stress is solved, there isn't any at all.

If for example, you have financial stress, don't work on the stress, work on your finances. If you have constant health stress, you get to work on your health. If you have stress over parenting, you work on your parenting.

From a more health focused perspective much of the world has been fixated on reducing stress through meditation and yoga and from a less healthy perspective with alcohol and comfort food. Hours are spent on stress reduction and avoiding stress, but has everyone forgotten about 'solving their problems?'

When I was $10,000 short on my bills, yoga or alcohol weren't going to stop the stress. At best, they would calm my nervous system and give me something to use as a distraction. Making the money reduced my stress. What is your stress and what are you doing to 'get the money?'

Worrying will never reduce your feelings of stress. Distracting yourself will not resolve it either. What can work well is solving the cause of the stress you have and if you cannot solve the whole thing in one go, take an action every day towards getting it done.

It took me 2 months to realise I wasn't even working on my financial stress. Once I did, I had peace again. What would happen if you worked though all of **your** stresses and got them complete?

2. Removing the Source of Stress

Removing the source of stress could involve, leaving that awful job, or not spending time with that energy-draining friend. You can't *solve* the job or the friend but you can let them go if they aren't adding value to your life.

Removing something, or someone from your life, can instantly take away stress. If you have a difficult work life, is it possible to leave the company, change positions, get promoted or work from home, work different hours, or change location?

What conversation could you have with your boss or clients?

I remember having a friend who was a regular stress in my life. I felt drained around him and wanted to be elsewhere when we were together. After agonising on what to do, I decided to move on from this friendship as it wasn't serving either of us.

I believe there is honour in 'letting people go,' that aren't fulfilling us. My former friend deserves someone who genuinely wants to be in his company. Afterwards, I'm happy to say he met new friends who do genuinely enjoy spending time with him.

Remember by staying in a situation you're not happy with, it is dishonouring all parties involved. You are stressed and neither are receiving exactly what is wanted and deserved. Every one of us deserve employment and people that match what we truly seek.

3. Changing Your Psychology: Self Talk

Let's start at the beginning with why thoughts occur. We all have thoughts and if you have just agreed or disagreed with that statement, that was a thought. We may have approximately 40,000-50,000 thoughts per day. Almost all of these thoughts, are 'thought' without you having to do any of the work.

The purpose of thoughts are to give feedback about our perception and environment. They let us know if we are safe, if the people in our life are loving and whether something is serving us or not. You can approach your thoughts, as feedback letting you know what is working and what is not working.

So, how can we use this to have a better relationship with our own mind? What can we do with stressful thoughts and emotions? One great shift in my life happened after reading a little yellow book by Joseph Murphy, called 'The Power of Your Subconscious Mind.'

The book taught me new approaches to successful self-talk and self-relating. I began approaching my mind like I would an actual relationship. Many of the things that make a person-to-person relationship work, can also be useful for self-relating.

Your subconscious mind has the great quality of acting with enthusiasm when given a task. It loves finding answers to questions (just as people do). If you are not currently giving your mind tasks for quitting addictions, stress reduction, or setting goals, you are wasting a valuable resource.

You could communicate with your mind in a variety of ways. You could ask it questions, treat it like a friend, demand results of it or in any way you choose. I have currently settled with treating my mind as I would a friend. I assume it is on my side and ask it questions for the betterment of my life. You could approach any relationship in your life with the qualities below and it will be effective.

- Asking for help.
- Giving compliments.
- Sticking to commitments.
- Being kind.
- Being quick to forgive.

I suggest you consider the little voice in your head as something you can relate to with inner communication. Will you start off communication with your subconscious mind like it is a friend, coach or perhaps higher power? It might start off a little awkwardly saying "hi" to your mind for the first time. Give it a go.

Your subconscious mind is a problem-solving resource that is awaiting your instructions.

Spend an hour conversing with your own mind. You have a wealth of wisdom inside you. Do this with a commitment to find an answer and it will prove a fruitful exercise. You could ask a question in the privacy of your own mind or you could write it down. As your subconscious mind gets used to this more direct way of communicating, you will accomplish a great deal.

Hold the idea that you will get the answers you need. Many times answers will come while you are chopping vegetables, driving a car, taking a shower or doing something similar. When focused intently on a task, your subconscious mind has space to solve problems.

Pronoia: The opposite of paranoia. The belief that your subconscious mind and life are conspiring in your favour.

In Review of Stress

We have explored how there is always something that can be done, when your level of stress is high. We discovered the difference between distracting from stress and actively solving problems. I no longer wish to be less stressed. When stress does arise I use 1 of the 3 approaches we chatted about. I work on taking purposeful action, rather than randomly reacting to my emotions.

We explored how to let go of stress that isn't working for you. It could be removing yourself from a damaging job or relationship. We discovered that most of our thoughts are automatic and that we have the ability to get our subconscious mind working for us, by asking it better questions.

When you are having a bad day (or year), don't spend too long avoiding worry. You can solve the problem, let go of the problem or use your mind to get answers you wouldn't otherwise have found.

Be careful not to use an addiction to alter how you feel. Using drugs or other addictions for this purpose, creates a dependence and coping mechanism. This means you will not develop strategies to deal with life. What we are doing here is opening you up to approaching stress from a position of power.

If you are in a bad mood or going through a tough time, avoid any type of substance or drug. In fact, on bad days you could look after yourself MORE, not less. You can support yourself mentally and physically through nearly anything.

Make a start here. Which of these would help lower your stress levels?

- Taking consistent action.
- Asking for help.
- Looking for gratitude in difficult situations.
- Getting grounded and being in nature.
- Service to others.
- Having fun.
- Quality food and exercise.
- Solving problems.
- Letting go of problems.
- Learn from what happened.

Parent Goals

An addiction is most likely to come back in the following scenarios. When there is extended time off work, a marriage breakdown, or someone close passes away. When you have a lot of high stress to deal with, the mind looks for an escape. It looks for a way to deal or not deal with emotions.

Use this time of transition to go for what you really want in life. The tides are shifting and this could be a very good time to decide which way you go. Maybe it's been a long time since you've thought of yourself. Perhaps there is something you would love to do, but have been holding back.

You may not feel like you are in a great mindset to set goals but this is precisely the best time to do it.

What is a parent goal then? A 'parent goal' is what I call a goal that gives you what you want AND eliminates problems along the way. A parent goal has big rewards and is deeply meaningful for you. It is a goal so meaningful, there is nothing that would stop you achieving it.

Parent Goals

The best demonstration of this is when a woman gets pregnant. 6/7 women (85.7%) stop or greatly reduce their compulsions and addictions as soon as they realise they are carrying a child. So too, do many of the men who are expecting to be fathers. The parents to-be have a purpose which keeps them inspired and on track.

Being a parent is an inspiring enough goal that addiction receptors in the brain literally turn off! The cravings from nicotine (supposedly one of the most addictive substances), disappears with pregnancy 85.7% of the time. The insight here for you, is to have something in your life to focus on, which inspires you enough to override lower impulses and cravings.

You are going through a time of change in life and I want you to dream big. Believe there are no limitations for you at all, no baggage to hold you back. You can have anything in life – what is it in your heart that you really want right now?

The potential rewards of a parent goal should be very high and fit in with who you are as a person. If naturally drawn to health, make it a health goal. If you are naturally drawn to spirituality, make it a spiritual goal and so on.

Having inspiring goals to work on, provides satisfaction in itself.

There is a difference between wishing for life not to be awful and setting goals to make your life successful and satisfying. I've created some demo parent goals that show how dreaming big, can be inspiring and take care of our stresses along the way.

- Don't wish you were out of debt... Set a goal to build a business or career that makes you millions of dollars, serves millions, allowing you to travel the world and enables you to become financially-free.

- Don't wish to save your marriage... Set a goal to have loving communication, regular touch & intimacy, connection, companionship, fun and enjoyment together.

- Don't wish to beat your compulsion or addiction... Set a goal to be free, happy, full of energy, motivated, living your purpose, exercising every day and loving life again.

So if you are looking to stop your compulsion or addiction, don't just wish to quit, find something that inspires you beyond all doubt to stay the course of sobriety. In the example above what I wish for also shows me the actions to help break the addiction. I can do things that make me feel free, happy and full of energy therefore I live my life around my purpose and exercise every day.

You will be much closer to achieving success with a parent goal that means something to YOU. It should be uniquely your own – something you would fight for (like a mother fights for her child)! Take 5 small or large action steps towards your goal every day. Do this for a year and you will have taken 1825 positive actions toward your goal.

I think I used to hope good things would just happen and granted sometimes they did. The difference now is, I am choosing what turns up in my life rather than getting dragged by the current and banging my head on life's proverbial rocks.

Fear

Fear is generated by our subconscious mind, assessing potential risk. Subconsciously when we believe an action will bring us more loss, than rewards, we hesitate. Every goal has fears that come along with it, otherwise everyone would be successfully taking action and achieving.

Whether your fears are rational or irrational, there are things you can do to overcome them. A parent goal is one of them.

If I get scared about a goal of my own of helping 10 million people, I focus on the value that other people will get. If I'm worried about my success, I'm just thinking about me and become nervous. If I'm focused on others, I'm being of service and all I think about is giving value. Fear does nothing, except to remind me to focus on others.

1) Remind yourself that fears are not facts, they are an assessment of risk. What are the chances of the fear surfacing? If it does happen, can you handle it? These questions are valuable to consider and steps can be taken to prepare for what could happen, so you are still playing the game of life.

2) Make your goal SO BIG that it overrides the fear response. Make your goal about serving other people. Working on something that is just for you isn't as powerful as doing something that impacts your family, community or the world.

Both men and women have an internal drive to achieve. We all have a part of us, active or inactive that wants to make a difference in the world. Inspiring goals are often easier to achieve because the payoff is highly attractive. **You are more likely to follow through with a goal you care about**.

The thing with a poorly worded goal is that it is demotivating. The language you use in your mind affects how likely you are to take action. Check out the difference between the ways these 2 goals are written. They are the same goal, but have a different energy about them.

Parent Goals

Option 1. I want to quit my addiction.

Option 2. I want to be free, happy, healthy, living my purpose serving others, exercising, feeling motivated and loving life again!

'Option 2' affirms what you want and ALSO reveals the path to get you there. Focus on finding what makes you happy & healthy, serving others, keeping fit and you get what you want while solving the problem. What you want, is the path.

I recommend that you set goals that take you beyond simply what you don't want and toward what you truly want to have. Setting a goal for $10 million, or serving 10 million people for example, is far more motivating than simply paying off your debts.

A parent goal takes care of the negative along the way and you will notice more opportunities than before.

The Easy Way to Be Disciplined

Are there ways to overcome self-sabotage and procrastination? Are there ways to be disciplined without having to use any willpower?

My secret to discipline is to not use willpower. It might sound strange but here is how it works. I don't wrestle with my own mind about whether to do something or not. I take actions that are in alignment with who I am based on what I am inspired by. Discipline comes from taking action that is in alignment with who you are.

I'm proposing that with a little shift in mindset, we can achieve goals without using large amounts of willpower. Sitting at a desk using technology for some is extremely difficult, for another, standing up, working outdoors all day will be equally difficult. Give these 2 people the job that matches their skills, personality traits and fitness levels and you'll have a much better match for who they are.

You can find those things in your life that are well suited to you. If you have to use lots of willpower in order to stay disciplined, it could be time to step back and examine why you are really doing, what it is you are doing. The reason self-sabotage exists may be to guide you back to something, that is better suited for you.

The distinction here is to take action based on what naturally inspires you, rather than from obligation. There are so many should dos and have tos in life that lead to exhaustion as opposed to feeling inspired by life... In the absence of inspiration, we often look for quick and easy fixes to **release us from pressure** or **a reward** to overcompensate for **giving too much**.

When I am working with a client and they've stated they "should quit smoking," or "should exercise," I know they have been using sheer willpower to make it happen. Making use of willpower doesn't lead to success, it leads to frustration and disappointment.

This links in with one of the central themes of this book. We do not condemn any behaviour by labelling it bad, we look at what is not working and adjust strategy. We look for the intention behind our old behaviour and seek alternatives that fit in better with our lifestyle and needs.

When you are living a life that is suited to your needs, you are likely to undergo a natural release of 'happy chemicals' in the brain, meaning you feel emotionally well and enjoy better sleep quality. If on the other hand you have a goal that is disappointing and frustrating you, consider these questions.

- Why do I have this goal?
- Is the goal actually for me, or someone else?
- What is an alternative that would work for me?
- Am I living my life based on inspiration or obligation?

Having a strong enough intention for your goals may help maintain discipline indefinitely. For a pregnant woman who is inspired to carry a healthy baby, her intention is strong, so she sticks to it. A goal with intention behind it creates stronger discipline.

Endeavour for an **intrinsic goal** which is something you naturally enjoy and find interesting. An **extrinsic goal** is motivated by external means and requires outside motivation and willpower or it is completed to avoid negative consequences. Try to avoid extrinsic goals because these are ones that produce only short term results.

This can be applied to healthy eating. You might change eating habits because your doctor told you to (extrinsic) or you genuinely enjoy the idea of looking after your body (intrinsic). Are you restricting certain foods and it's a battle (extrinsic)? Or are you eating better because your focus is on loving your body (intrinsic)?

If the intention is being on a short term diet to lose weight, your goal is extrinsic. It may not be possible to lose weight every week AND if your food plan is short term and you lose weight, what is the plan for after the diet?

Most people return to their original eating habits once the motivation of a diet wears off. So, don't diet. Eat food that you **love** and is **good for your body**. Eat food that **satisfies you** and helps you **lose weight**. Be **consistent** but not over the top. Eat great, **nutritious food 90% of the time** and be **flexible**.

The cycle of losing and re-gaining weight is a result of extrinsic thinking. Trying to just get a result. "I should lose weight, so I should exercise. I should eat better. I should, I should, I should." Many of the clients I see are very stressed about food and are trying hard, but are frustrated and disappointed by results.

They are stressed because they have restricted foods and are exercising in ways they don't love (or even like). Restriction of any food, leads to a case of overeating later on. We need a better plan for our families and society. Using intrinsic goals gives one inner rewards that one could stick to forever.

The effort becomes not battling with the old, but building the new.

I apply the use of intrinsic goals to my addiction process when working with people. We work together towards never having to use willpower again (wherever possible) and focus additionally on what they get from their habit or addiction and how to satisfy core needs from healthy sources.

Telling someone their addition is bad doesn't help them quit, we know this. Finding out what their needs are and how to satisfy them is a surer path to recovery. You can apply this very reasoning to anything *you* no longer wish to do. Examine what you get from an old behaviour and find means to satisfy that from things you enjoy.

Coming Home

Author Elizabeth Gilbert talks about how experiencing great rejection and great success can both be difficult, as it can take us away from what we love. She talks about how returning to your vocation (what you love) can bring you back home in your heart.

When her best seller, 'Eat Pray Love' found success, she was swept up in praise and interviews but quickly felt disconnected. She returned to her writing and felt home. When her next book 'Committed' bombed, she was swept up in criticism and interviews, leaving her disconnected. She returned to writing and felt home.

The gaining of praise and avoiding criticism from others is not the goal of life. Doing what you love because it feels like home, just might be.

My 'home' is in helping people be free from addiction, anxiety and depression. I savour a 30-40 year problem a person may have and guiding their release from it. I do it when I have a day off and on holidays, I did it in Egypt crossing the Nile River. You don't need days off when you love what you do.

If you aren't currently doing exactly what you love, draw up a list as big as you can of everything you enjoy. Write down things you love to do without ever having to be asked. Include things that interest you and things you deny yourself because you think they're silly or taboo. Keep going until you have 100+ things written down. Your 'home' is somewhere there.

If Elizabeth tried to recreate the feelings of success from her first book, that would be an extrinsic goal. Writing a book on a topic she is fascinated by, would be intrinsic. It doesn't feel like work when it's an intrinsic goal. It would come naturally to her as it would you because you are inspired from within.

In Review:

- Choose actions that are truly in alignment with who you are.
- Let go of things that don't match your authentic self.
- Intrinsic goals are long lasting and don't rely on merely gaining pleasure and avoiding pain.
- Don't use willpower to change a habit, search inside for a deeper intention that serves love.

Remember, the next time you are using willpower to stay disciplined, ask yourself, what is the purpose? Start taking actions that are good for you and you are also inspired by and in doing this you won't stop when things start to get difficult. You'll keep going.

I hope these ideas provide you with new ways to approach discipline to improve results and personal satisfaction.

Food: The Most Complicated Addiction

We all eat for different reasons and food has a unique effect on people. Some put on weight easily whilst others seem to eat 'anything' and their weight remains consistent.

There is a varying affect foods and drinks have on our energy levels too. For some, certain food types will increase energy and for others, it will drain it. You are a unique individual and it will be your own unique food plan that works best.

When working on your health, NEVER compare your situation to another. Do not buy into someone else's journey if it doesn't actually fit in with your life and your body. What works for one person, may not necessarily work for you, and vice-versa.

One of my relatives can eat steak and drink coffee, within 30 minutes of going to bed and have no sleep problems however for most, this would mean being awake half the night bloated and feeling lethargic the next day. We wouldn't follow his sleep plan, just because it works for him. Likewise, we wouldn't follow someone's bizarre diet just because it worked for them.

We'll talk about finding a food plan that works for you in this chapter. That means consuming food in a way that adds quality to your experience of life and yourself. The result of what you eat should not take away from feelings of well-being, energy levels, or how you feel about yourself.

Look for a combination of what is science based and works best for you.

Avoid stories in magazines with sensationalist type headlines. These stories give contrary advice for health, purely for the purpose of getting attention which is steered toward increasing sales. The set intention is not geared for your health and articles of this nature tend to misguide those who are most desperate to lose weight and get healthy. Ironically, it is these very people who are the ones in most need of quality advice.

I have spotted a magazine article that stated, "you don't need water to lose weight." Another article had the headline, "why you need cake to lose weight." When creating *your* relationship with food, take your advice from the highest sources you can.

During the time I spent healing myself, I had read 1100 books on health, healing and human behaviour. Common points on health and weight loss unfolded after much reading as I observed methods that have stood the test of time which do not require a 'junk' headline to sell it.

The process of finally turning my own health around entailed my reading of several hundred books and attending a dozen trainings in mind-body health, only to find the effectiveness in hearing the same message over and over again in order to change my actions. I've deliberated that perhaps change takes time and each step builds upon the last.

Beyond silly magazine articles and morning show programs are detailed studies into health and weight loss and I have gathered these resources together because I believe they will give you the best chance of finding a successful food plan.

Why you put on weight and precisely what foods to eat sourced by the Mudita Institute:

https://inspirehypnotherapy.com/2018/03/weight-loss

One of the largest studies into human nutrition sourced by The China Study:

https://inspirehypnotherapy.com/2018/04/the-china-study

How to stop emotional eating and lose weight:

https://inspirehypnotherapy.com/2015/09/achieve-your-ideal-weight

Test Your Way to Success

A valuable way to approach change is to get good at testing new ideas. It took me a few years of gradual improvement in getting my food plan close to 100% right for me. I packed my plate with real foods. Real foods are those that grow, have their own outer casing or need to be peeled.

I conducted a small survey of 25 people who gave up all sugar (except fruit) for one week or longer.

- 72% of people said they had a moderate to large increase in energy.
- 16% of people said there was no difference or a small increase in energy.
- 12% of people said they had a decrease in energy.

I tested the effectiveness of quitting sugar, wheat, dairy and red meat for 2 weeks in 2012. My energy had more than doubled and I stopped experiencing any energy loss in the afternoons. After 4 years of fatigue this was the biggest healing step I undertook. Food cravings disappeared. Pain in my body decreased. I felt alive. 7 years on and those food items are a negligible part of my diet.

Be an expert at learning, not at knowing everything there is to know.

The word 'expert' has its origin in Latin. One of the early definitions is, "a person wise through experience." We don't become wise unless we test something new and expand our experience. Anything that works well for you, can be kept as a part of your permanent lifestyle.

It may be valuable for you to eat more real foods (foods that grow) and minimise heavy and processed foods for a period of time. Test what is possible for your body by eating lightly and taking the pressure off your digestion system.

The Most Complicated Addiction

Psychologically, food may have the largest number of positive and negative associations, of any compulsion or addiction. It is in the top 5 things we do most as human beings, amongst breathing, blinking, sleeping and body movement.

Unlike other habits, we never get rid of food. It will always remain part of our lives, because we won't ever 'quit' food as we might drugs, the solution must include relating to it in a healthy way. We want food to be a positive part of our life.

In this chapter I'm going to use the words **healthy** and **unhealthy** loosely. The intention is to promote freedom from food issues, not judgement. In order to discuss food we would need the use of words. Neither healthy nor unhealthy have anything to do with good or bad and right or wrong. They are to represent what is **working** and **not working** for human beings in our relationship with food.

With that being said, let's explore food together. Our relationship with food goes far deeper than we might expect. Working with clients on their habits, travelling overseas and having been part of a family myself, have shown me how differently we all eat.

Why We Eat

There is what could be called healthy eating. This might include: eating when hungry, eating for the purposes of receiving nutrition, eating real foods, enjoying flavours and textures of food, feeling satisfied after a meal, consuming food in order to fuel up and to boost your immune function.

Unhealthy eating could include: eating in overly large portions, eating just before sleep, binge eating, feeling very restricted with food choices, stress eating, obsessed with or repelled by food, eating to change your emotions, eating mainly processed foods.

Let's examine here the main reasons 'overeating' and 'stress eating' occurs. Is the reason you do it, one of these listed here?

- To feel comfort.
- To reward yourself.
- Because you just enjoy it.
- Because you have difficulty saying "no" when offered food.
- Because it is quick and easy.
- Because you are rebelling against someone/something.
- Because everyone else is and you don't want to miss out.

Working out why you eat the way you do, can

provide you with a starting point to transform yourself if you have non-functional eating habits.

We can explore a few more questions about our food choices: Is it something I do because I was raised that way? Are my eating habits making me feel alive? Is that behaviour working or not working right now? With this knowledge, what new choices can I make today?

In the process of writing this chapter, I abstained from all sugar, except that derived from fruit for 7 days. This is something I do periodically to reset my mind if sugar creeps back into my diet. During the week that I abstained from sugar, I had an average of 10 cravings a day. Most cravings were weak, while some were much stronger. Every time I had a craving, I took an alternate action instead of giving in it.

I paid close attention to how I was *feeling* at times I experienced cravings. The 2 biggest cravings occurred when I felt disappointed. I wasn't looking for sugar at all, I was looking to feel better! There are hundreds of ways to feel better that are also good for me.

I did not use willpower to resist the cravings, I observed them for a moment before acting. I asked myself, "What do I really need right now?" This is a communication strategy you can use with your own mind (similar to the one we discussed in the Dealing with Stress chapter of this book). I am receiving the answer for what will completely satisfy the craving.

As I hadn't immediately acted on every craving, I found a variety of hidden needs. Sometimes I was thirsty for water, on occasion it was time for a normal meal so I ate anyway. Still other times I was emotional and focused on dealing with the problem at hand.

The urge to ingest sugar was very strong when anxiety and disappointment arose.

You're not alone if you use food to change how you feel. Everyone has done it. We've all snacked or devoured too much because we were emotional. It is often the quickest and easiest solution perceived at the time. With that being said, freedom from those cravings can be gained by finding better ways to deal with emotions.

If your primary way to deal with stress, is to eat or drink, then there is a fair chance you are avoiding an ongoing issue in your life. Emotions are no good reason to eat unhealthily. Food can never satisfy emotions.

Food and People

Food is social, which means there can be expectations from others about HOW you eat. You may be eating too much, or too little, because that's the way your family always have. In some families you are 'expected' to eat unhealthily, at times of festivity like: Christmas, Easter, birthdays, holidays, weddings, or simply because it's the weekend.

The pressure to eat like the people you spend time with is real. It is not spoken about directly, but it exists. What are the eating habits of the 5 people you spend the most time with? What do they partake of? How much? If you follow their lead this may be a determining factor in your own outcome of health.

One of my first weight loss clients, Jodie, created a nice strategy for turning down foods that she was offered from her husband... After dinner he would always bring her food she didn't want. Chips, crackers, cheese, salami and more alcohol. Time after time he would offer her something extra and she would say, "thank you for thinking of me" and get a glass of water.

She utilised his offer of heavy food as a reminder to herself to drink water (this is genius, because she wins twice using the one strategy, avoiding unwanted foods and drinking more water instead). Remember there is nothing 'wrong' with cheese, salamis and alcohol. For Jodie, these just weren't fitting in with the results she wanted for her body.

Rather than feeling guilty (the number 1 emotion to clear when working on weight loss) in turning down food from loved ones, she found a way to powerfully look after herself and her relationship. He gets a thank you for thinking of her and she gets to feel healthy and comfortable in her body again!

Parental Rules

There can be pressure from parental figures to eat in a certain way. Lines such as, "finish everything on your plate, or else no dessert for you," are **highly confusing** when you think about it. Here we have parents forcing children to eat healthy food --> so they can freely give them unhealthy food as a reward.

Read that twice.

The 'food rules' parents create, often are to encourage children to partake of vegetables or something similar. Rules from parents though, can make food confusing.

The problem here is, these kids are growing into adults and rewarding themselves with junk food. This faulty reward system leaves them feeling stressed and guilty, because they know it's not working for the body.

Why is sugar considered a treat anyway? 150 years ago sugar was linked with being of wealth and high social status. To get a hold of sugar back then was a real treat. Are there alternative ways you can reward your kids that do not include sugar? Affection, praise, reading them a story, or playing games are a few possibilities.

Food should not be our main reward system or used daily for that purpose.

Another common reason for eating more than we know is good for us, is to not waste food. The 'story' is that we should not waste food because there are children who are starving in other parts of the world. In reality, whether we consume or not, the other person still doesn't get any.

Part of a solution to stop eating beyond what we need, is to serve in a smaller bowl of food to begin with. It gives us a feeling of completion after a meal. We can store any remaining cooked food for another time. These steps take care of you and avoids having to waste or over-consume.

Food and Body Image

Food can be deeply associated with body image and body image can be linked with identity. If how we eat is linked to the shape of our body, then food, the humble stuff that keeps us alive, becomes linked with guilt and shame about who we are.

I had dysfunctional eating patterns for more than half of my life. My earliest memory of having stress with food came at 12 years old. Devouring large amounts so people wouldn't assume I was under-eating. I had overheard the word anorexic a few times and I was determined not to be spoken of in relation to that.

Being a skinny kid brought the fear that others assumed I suffered from anorexia or bulimia. I recall being scared and delaying a visit to the bathroom straight after dinner mainly to prevent people thinking I was throwing my food up. I spent a great amount of mental energy controlling how others viewed me. It was tiring.

I ate chocolate or sugar in some form every day for 20 years. I thought I needed it. Again I would sometimes have more than I even wanted making certain I didn't get skinnier. I longed for the day when others thought my slight frame a mark of genetics, rather than behaviour.

These days I accept myself the way I am. My body is fantastic in hundreds of ways, skinny or a bit bulkier. I love the way it looks, feels, keeps me warm, the way it provides symptoms if fed something incompatible, the sheer joy and pleasure it gives, range of movement, its ability to laugh and love and a range of other things it allows me to experience.

Symptoms in the body are feedback letting me know conditions in my life are not compatible for well-being. Symptoms such as self-guilt and frustration are a reminder to take action and correct something that is not working. Symptoms are feedback.

There is pressure on both women and men to look a certain way and plenty of skinny shaming to go along with overweight shaming. There is nothing wrong with any Body. Every shape and size is worthy of feeling comfortable in and loved. Your body is worthy of love.

I want you to keep in mind that your body is not your identity. You are not skinny, you are not fat, you are not a size 6, and you are not a size 18. Your body has a shape and size and that is not WHO you are. You HAVE a body and it is wonderful in many ways.

The way your body appears to you is not your identity. Your identity is not how you eat or a particular size. Identity is made up of all the wonderful parts of you: intelligence, creativity, career, role in family, skills, nationality, friendships, and your contribution to others, your faith and compassion.

Let your identity include every wonderful part of you, not just the part you are challenged by. Your identity is all of who you are. Take note of what you say to yourself after the words "I am." Make those words after "I am" something beautiful about yourself!

The Big Secret about Guilt

There was a lady I worked with in late 2015, named Vicky. She was 50 years old and working on quitting smoking. She started to talk about her health and family situation. She was struggling with her health and not getting the respect she wanted from her daughter. Through the course of our conversation she shared that she truly would not care if death came to her.

At the time there was not much point in us talking about health benefits of quitting smoking. Instead, I suggested she write a short list of 50 ways in which she is a magnificent person. Tension rose (I expected it would) as I had directly presumed that she certainly is magnificent and a mere 50 points is a short list in getting us started on proving it. After a short time she simply declared that there was nothing great about her.

Any person who tells you they are not magnificent is lying to you. Don't believe them.

It is not possible for someone to be alive for 50 years, assist people through careers, raise a family and be a human being without having worth. She was stuck in an identity of not being good enough. A way forward from there is to recall every time you were good enough, up until tears appear in your eyes and you feel gratitude in your heart.

Previously, Vicky had proficiently worked as an accountant, saving clients hundreds of thousands of dollars and was at the time caring for her daughter and granddaughter in her home. She was more giving than most and accomplished a great many things in life but a negative mindset had taken hold, denying access to self-worth.

Vicky had an immensely low opinion of herself but that was not the truth. Our session continued to reveal 8 ways that she believed she was magnificent. It being quite a feat in digging to get those 8! I noted she had opened the door to seeing that she had at least some greatness.

Shame is a mask covering over your achievements and magnificence.

You may recall from the stress chapter, that stress has a purpose behind it. Rather than wishing the stress away, we saw there are steps that could be taken by anyone. The same is true for guilt and shame. These emotions have a purpose behind them and there is something you can do about it. You are not stuck.

The secret of guilt is to show there are thoughts you **believe about yourself that aren't true and things you are not appreciating**. It's not about feeling bad but the guilt letting you know there is something important, that needs your personal reflection. The guilt is doing its job.

What can be done to shift your beliefs? How do you stop feeling ashamed or guilty? You stop pretending that you aren't worthwhile. It takes vulnerability and risking being hurt again. When you take a risk, you open the door to live joyfully, powerfully and free again. You are wonderful. Own it.

No one can be a human being and not have a value.

Write a small list of 50-100 things about yourself that are magnificent. Ask others to contribute to get you started. Include things you love about yourself and ways that you have helped people, until you feel your energy shift.

The Guilt and Dieting Cycle

- You restrict food with a diet to lose weight.
- You do well for a short time.

The Big Secret About Guilt

- You have a bad day and eat the foods you previously restricted.
- You feel a release from stress, then overindulge.
- You feel guilty and think, "Why bother, I'll eat what I want."
- You do that and feel guiltier.
- Food becomes a 'buffer' against failure now. If you're not trying any more, you can't fail and get hurt!
- You are trapped eating in ways that don't serve you and are afraid to try once more.
- Your symptoms of discomfort and guilt increase and eventually you diet again.

The typical diet is a strategy to eat smaller amounts of foods or cut out certain foods in order to lose weight. An opportunity to exit the dieting cycle is to make your 'diet' a long term food plan that has nothing to do with restriction. Restriction is using willpower. That leads to an over-consumption after several weeks or months.

The food plan should not be a 'diet' at all. It should work and also be one that you feel you could follow forever.

In Conclusion: What Healthy Eating Looks Like

Healthy eating consists of not restricting or overindulging. It is a balanced approach to food. A balanced approach is something that works for you (does not produce body symptoms, like reflux, diabetes, guilt etc.) and it is easy to commit to because it feels natural.

Eventually, a food plan of your choice will work for your body and lifestyle. Base food choices on the best information you can and make small changes over time. Avoid the latest fad diet and give your body what it is truly looking for most of the time – water and real foods.

1) How much you eat: The amount of food you eat is one of the obvious ones to get right. Eating above required quantity puts organs under constant stress in having to digest as much, which in turn leaves you lethargic. Serving portion sizes too small leaves one unsatisfied.

Generally it is better to eat 3-5 smaller meals per day, as opposed to 1 or 2 big meals.

2) What you eat: The type of food you eat can help balance your weight, emotions and energy levels. Go for light foods that are easier to digest. It may be wise to reduce the quantity of heavy and processed food types, including: meat, dairy, wheat, white potatoes and processed sugar. Consume real foods and avoid processed foods.

Real food grows and processed food generally comes in a packet.

3) When you eat: The first hour of the day is an apt time for when you can improve health and weight loss results. For the first hour of each day, choose some or all of these activities to make up your morning ritual.

i) Walk before breakfast.

ii) Drink warm water with lemon.

iii) Have breakfast.

iv) Meditation.

v) Write a to-do list for the day.

Start your day powerfully and you will live powerfully.

4) Avoid emotional eating: If how you eat changes based on your mood, to some degree this is considered emotional eating. Find positive ways to reduce stress and worry, which have nothing to do with food or alcohol. Nurture yourself a little once a day and a lot once a week.

Don't let eating to change how you feel, become a habit.

5) Be consistent: Select a food plan you are certain you could follow for years. Avoid any food plan that involves too much restriction. Eat well 90% of the time and allow yourself to have a bad day or week. Release the need to be perfect.

Eat well 90% of the time and let go of all the pressure and guilt you've been carrying.

6) Eat consciously: When you catch yourself going to the cupboard when bored, make a decision in accordance with this question. "What do I really want right now?" Take a new action based on what you require. Can you find something else to equally satisfy you? A glass of water or something productive may suffice.

Eat in awareness, not just because you are bored or stressed.

False Cravings

I wonder how often the craving for something unhealthy, is actually a craving for something else. Stay with me here. This is an expansion on the idea that we aren't looking for the addiction itself, we are looking for what it *does* for us. Granted we have needs however there are a variety of things that can satisfy us.

There were instances where I have opened kitchen cupboards in search of snacks, even though I wasn't hungry. On a date I have eaten extra at a restaurant wanting not to appear wasteful. I've chosen food that I normally wouldn't have, to make a partner happy.

I am proposing that the human body does not crave anything that is bad for it. What the body is actually craving are hidden needs that you are becoming aware of. In examples above, opening the kitchen cupboards satisfied the need of **relief from boredom**. I ate extra **not to appear wasteful to others**. I ate what I hadn't wanted to **please a partner**.

You don't consciously make these types of decisions, these are automatic responses made by the subconscious mind. The purpose of being aware of your hidden needs are simply to be aware of them. When you discover what your needs are, you can make a more purposeful choice.

I am theorising that all cravings are false cravings, because they can be satisfied by something other than the addiction or compulsion.

A sugar craving can be another example of a false craving. Those who experience higher rates of sugar cravings are lacking in Chromium and Magnesium. The body appears to crave sugar but when vitamins are taken, they no longer crave sugar as much and cravings often diminish.

A lady I worked with in 2014 consumed 2L of sugary drinks a day and generally snacked unhealthily. Within a 24 hour period of taking these vitamins, her sugar consumption went from 2L a day, down to one small glass of Pepsi and she'd cut out all the extra snacking.

Another common false craving would be nicotine in cigarettes. When I smoked my very last cigarette, I knew I wasn't craving nicotine! I was out with a couple of cute girls at a night club and they were smoking, so I did too, in order to get closer to them. That's not nicotine, that's looking for connection.

False Cravings

I've questioned 1100 smokers on their reason for starting again after quitting previously. Every single person reported to have had a really bad day, or simply "just had one" when socialising or drinking. Every person who started smoking again after giving it up for 1 week or longer, did so for reasons other than nicotine. They did it to **feel better** or **connect** with people.

Your Brain Can Turn Off Cravings

I've heard it said more than a few times that nicotine is the hardest substance to quit. Is it a nicotine craving or associations such as stress relief that you connect with a smoking habit? Here is observational evidence that nicotine may not be as addictive as you first thought.

1) You sleep through 6-8 hours without smoking every night but need a cigarette every 30 minutes during the day. Your brain automatically knows how to turn off a craving when you're asleep or whenever you are highly occupied throughout the day.

2) Many people who smoke tell me they are able to take a 12 hour flight or engage in activities all day and not receive a single craving. Some smoke none at home with family and copiously when at work. This has little to do with nicotine and more to do with how the person feels in their workplace.

3) 6/7 women quit cigarettes as soon as they receive news of their pregnancy. It could be that carrying a healthy baby is important or that it would be embarrassing to smoke and be pregnant, that helps them quit. The significance of something meaningful helps one to free themselves from addiction.

Your brain has the ability to turn off cravings under the right conditions. For a mother to be, cigarettes are no longer an addiction and are deemed rather impossible. There are more to cravings than just physical dependence on nicotine.

Granted, some may have to deal with nicotine withdrawal, however when you deal with associations to cigarettes, these cravings become less and pass much quicker – your needs are being met. Here are the top 5 triggers that turn up for the cigarette smokers I see. A false craving for nicotine is often about how they associate cigarettes with these things.

1. Stress.
2. Boredom.
3. Socialising.
4. With coffee.
5. A substitute for eating/ keeping weight reduced.

Below are more general examples that give you an idea about what may be behind your cravings. The purchasing of shoes for example, is not a substance like cigarettes which is consumed by your body, yet you experience a craving like you would a physical addiction.

- False craving for buying shoes can = looking for validation, a treat, or a self-esteem boost.
- False craving for nicotine can = looking to feel better, relax, or socialise.
- False craving for comfort food can = looking for a reward, sweetness, or comfort.
- False craving for alcohol can = needing to shut off the mind.

Cravings always have content behind them. In the **WARP** we will go in depth on alternatives for reducing cravings so you can be free from addiction.

A subconscious mind *doesn't know* about false cravings, it knows that your compulsion or addiction seems to be the quickest way to satisfy some of your wants and needs. Your subconscious mind isn't well equipped at breaking long-term compulsions without intervention.

We know there are behaviours that disadvantage us. When in the midst of an addiction we are not able to see consequences, or the many things that can give us an equal satisfaction. This will be our mission. A discovery of your hidden needs and retraining your mind to satisfy those in a better way.

An addiction is most likely to return when you have work stress, a marriage breakdown, or someone close to you passes away. When you have high levels of stress to deal with, the mind looks for escape and a way to deal, or not deal with emotions.

When thoughts stray to giving up on your goal of being addiction free, don't let those thoughts win! Observe and take a different action instead. A measure of self-mastery is the degree to which you observe thoughts without needing to immediately act on them.

Observe your thoughts without the need to act on them.

Thoughts you may have, such as, "it's okay I'll just do it once more," "I'll quit next month when the time is right," or "we've all got to go (die) in some way," are not thought patterns that are increasing your personal power. Thoughts like these do not appear on purpose but you are the one who decides whether to act on them. Take actions on thoughts that make you better.

Turn Doubts into Success

At the Beijing Olympics of 2008 Michael Phelps achieved a total of 8 gold medals, the most ever in any single Olympic game. During his 8th race his goggles began to fill with water but Michael didn't miss a stroke. He succeeded 7 elite athletes because he had trained for anything that could possibly go wrong, hundreds of times over.

The doubt and worry of his goggles filling with water was replaced by confidence in knowing it wouldn't matter because he was prepared for it. Here is a very nice example of having doubts then **making yourself better**. He was the best in the world because he took doubt and increased his ability to respond to it.

In the course of accomplishing your goals, you will have feelings of both confidence and doubt. When a doubt comes up, observe it and thank it for reminding you how far you've come. Don't resist the doubt. Notice it and take an empowered action in the opposite direction instead.

I tend to treat my doubts like a friend inviting me to be better. From this perspective, I can always win! When I doubt, I reflect on whether I have room to improve my words and actions. I always do. I can work on being better one action at a time.

Turn Doubts into Success

For example, had I doubts on stopping an addiction, I would reflect on what's necessary in making sure I am successful. Who can be counted on for support? Can I plan better this time? Which people will it benefit me to avoid? Can I better support my body in recovery with food and exercise? Do I have a plan to deal with stress and loneliness? What else do I need to be successful?

Make a plan based on these questions and ready yourself for inevitable challenges. Improve the quality of your planning and actions. Doubts can make you better, that's why they are there. Doubt lets you know that **a plan to quit your addiction, needs strength behind it**. Don't wish doubt would go away, improve yourself and seek support in beating it.

My Journey to Mastery

Mastery, to be responsible for creating one's own life experience. The ability to decide one's own path. Skill in handling difficult: thoughts, emotions, habits and addictions. Mastery is not perfection. Mastery is freedom to choose. The choosing of what best serves ourselves and others. Mastery is action. There is time for reflection and letting the mind still. Stillness occurs only when there is no more action to carry out. Mastery is acting on higher thoughts and learning from lower, or base thoughts.

Chronic fatigue had set in from 2008 – 2012. I felt everyday what it was like to be tired, weak, anxious and sore. Bearing acute pain upon waking as if been hit by a truck in my sleep. I was driven to discover what it took to be an empowered, healthy individual.

The following foundations of health are presently what I do every day. These foundations support both the mind and body for optimal health, strengthening immune function and well-being. Without them you may be missing the most vital ingredients for health and healing.

I use these for several applications including: physical health, boosting of energy levels and stress reduction. **A gradual or possibly immediate turn for your health are likely and will ensure much difference**.

You can support your body and mind through temporary symptoms to become well.

The '7 Cornerstones of Amazing Health' have no side-effects. They contain no downsides. Don't be fooled by their simplicity. When you get these working at the right level, it's really hard to not become healthy.

1) Breathe deeply. As you settle the rhythm of your breathing, your emotional state starts to match that rhythm. We are panicky, emotional, or agitated when a craving develops, our breath has the ability to settle emotions and our mind. **Breathe steadily and continuously for 10 minutes** and you will change how you feel. Practise until you reach mastery.

2) Drink Water. Water is the second most essential nutrient for your body, after oxygen. Keeping hydrated means more oxygen is carried through your circulation system, which positively impacts your brain and vital organs. When you are well hydrated you think clearly and experience **less instances of cravings because your body is getting what it actually needs**.

3) Eat Real Food. Repairing your relationship with food is crucial when transforming an addiction or compulsion. **The most highly stressed people** I have worked with, have the most disordered relationships with food. When abandoning an addiction, eating well is amongst the top things you must do to recover.

4) Exercise is useful as a replacement behaviour from addiction. Exercise is one of the few activities that render **massive highs and is good for you**, physically and mentally. Body movement that gets you sweating, increases your heart rate and orders your body to grow stronger.

5) Being Still. Resting of your body and mind, through activities like meditation, is a form of honouring self. **Being still for 20 minutes or longer activates the parasympathetic nervous system**. This reduces blood pressure, relaxes organs, improves digestion and restores the body.

6) Self-Talk. Human beings converse with ourselves as well as each other. Consider how often your mind is talking about what you don't want, versus what you do want. **Set goals of positive affirmation** and remind yourself to be grateful every day.

7) Purpose. A purpose is something you have a strong inclination toward. It could be something you are

already doing or have resisted for a long while. **Purpose makes you come alive, energises and fills you up inside.** Dedicate yourself to that and you won't have time to waste on an old addiction, any more.

Health is an automatic response to your body receiving what it *truly* needs. The '7 Cornerstones of Amazing Health' are all free and every one of these can be implemented daily. How many boxes out of 7 can you currently tick? Is there 1 or more missing from your health plan right now?

Pain and Drugs

Addiction could seem like an option in times of great pain, divorce, losing a family member or loss of career. Intense pain may fuel a belief that you won't get through it. There is a need for: perspective, support, love and time to process all that is happening.

Learning how to better deal with pain will be an enormous part of your freedom from addiction journey. Like stress, pain lets you know there is something that needs your attention. The more pain is ignored, the louder it gets. Pain has a voice that is asking to be heard.

It is crucial not to associate an addiction with pain relief, if you do then the more pain you experience the more you will use something damaging in an attempt to relieve it. Pain is not meant to be suppressed indefinitely, it is something that has to be gone through in order to fully process. Seek support at times of physical and emotional pain.

Pain is related to some form of gain and loss. We receive pain for we have gained something terrible or lost something we perceived as valuable. Gaining a chronic disease is an example of something terrible.

Losing a loved one could be an example of losing something valuable.

Case Study Wendy

Wendy had been admitted to hospital after constant thoughts of self-harm and nightmares in which she cut her own neck. She revealed she had no intention of hurting herself but thoughts were overwhelming. She had been prescribed anti-depressant medication and come to see me because the nightmares were persisting.

Wendy was in her late twenties and had fallen in love with her older ex-boss, Chris. He made it abundantly clear that he did not want a relationship by filing a workplace harassment complaint about her. Despite this rejection she continued to believe that they would marry one day. Her feelings of withdrawal from Chris were no different to what a drug user would experience.

Fantasies of pleasure with no pain can drive addictive behaviour.

She was dealing with intense anger towards him and self. The pain was mentally and physically overwhelming. Wendy wished the pain would just go away! She tried pushing it out of her mind, but it pushed back!

I shared with her that marrying the gentleman or not, should be secondary to her wellbeing (after all when we are empowered, we stand the best chance of attracting a quality mate). We created a self-care ritual for her that would involve: weekly hypnotherapy, breath work, hydration, quality food, yoga, meditation, daily gratitude, time with friends and taking action on her career plans.

I asked her questions about the qualities she most wanted in a husband, character traits Chris displayed and the reality of who she really was. When I asked about what she wanted in a mate, it was nothing like how she described Chris. It was my intention she discover this difference on her own, rather than give her advice.

In my opinion the pain was letting her know, she was holding onto something that was not real. Chris was actually not a match, or even interested in marriage. It would not have been okay for me to say that directly though, as she was already judging herself harshly. My function was to ask questions that bring about realisations of truth.

By her third appointment, Wendy's pain was substantially reduced and her mental clarity returned. Her nightmares had reduced from every night to just once over the week since our last meeting. The combination of breaking the fantasy relationship and her self-care ritual, supported her to become balanced.

When we assume that pain has a purpose, we can approach it from a position of power. It is letting us know that something is out of balance – we want something different than what life gives us! Pain lets us know to change conditions. This means changing our physical conditions and mental perspective.

What Pain Wants From You

1) Pain wants you to listen. It is feedback, letting you know something in life needs attention. If you ignore pain, it loudly retaliates. If you drown it, guess what, it knows how to swim. Giving attention to pain helps us understand its purpose and what we can potentially do about it.

2) Pain wants action. It acts to inform us where something little or great is not working. Don't blame pain for doing its job, without it, we would be lack vital feedback about what we need. Taking action on your pain is a process that takes time. This remains a safer option than using addictions for temporary relief.

The action for **emotional pain** could be to let go of grief or anger you have been carrying. The action for **physical pain** could be changing how you move your body, stretching and treatment to allay discomfort.

For loneliness it could be finding something or someone to connect with again in areas of self, friends, family, community, nature or spiritual.

3) Pain wants to be appreciated. This one will take some inner work. Pain has its place. I am grateful that my own pain lets me know which foods are incompatible, when people aren't good for me and it forces me to take new action when something isn't working in relationships.

The next pain you encounter, don't *just* wish it away, spend time reflecting on the meaning of your pain. What is the message? Pain has your interests at heart after all. It gives you guidance to be more at ease with your life. Take actions to reduce the source of your pain and find things to appreciate about your difficult situation.

Good Day Vs Bad Day

After 2000 sessions as a hypnotherapist, patterns have emerged about how people approach stress and painful experiences. Doing something unhealthy whenever things went wrong seem to be the norm for many. They had little belief in changing circumstances, so they avoided what was going on.

In Australia and in Western culture the need for a 'beer' or 'wine' after a long day is observable. We pursue the fastest, easiest way to relax and avoid problems on our mind. The need to relax could display itself as problem drinking, smoking cigarettes and stress eating. These fit distracting and unhealthy criteria. They are also legal.

Noticeably on bad days people tend to look after themselves less. It has been a mission of mine to turn this mindset around. A 180 degree turn can be taken on bad days. **When having a rough day, take the approach of looking after yourself.** Shifting your mindset away from unhealthy to healthy habits to feel better. Shouldn't this be the go-to approach for us all?

The philosophy I encourage is to use the '7 Cornerstones of Amazing Health' on bad days as a first resort. Over time your body lets go of seeking addiction for relief. Find healthy options to change how you feel, that work, so you don't become dependent on an unhealthy something to feel good.

On tough days we don't feel like doing something healthy and boring... but this is precisely the time we need it.

Use stress as a signal, to look after yourself more. You can turn self-sabotage around by thinking about what your body needs the most when it is stressed. **It might need support.** You don't need to make a perfect decision every day, but aim to make quality ones most of the time. Rather than avoiding stress, set a long term goal to sort out issues behind it.

Affirmation: "During difficult times, I take action on what I can, appreciate what I can't change and support my body and mind to get through it."

Caution with Medications

There are reasons why depression and anxiety exist. Pain always has content behind it. In each case there are a combination of issues that may need to be worked on and through to transform.

I would support the position of using medication to deal with emotions, as a last resort. My reasoning behind this is a belief in fixing problems, rather than fixing emotions. After all, emotions are feedback *about* the problem. An avoidance of problems is detrimental as seen through observation of clients.

Let's use 'receiving an email' to your inbox, as a way to illustrate your emotional feedback system. In this analogy the email is emotion delivered to you by your subconscious mind. Emotions send you information.

What is inside the email is the content. The content of an email could state for example, that you have a large financial debt. Now it is not useful to be upset

Pain and Drugs

with emails (the delivery system) and try to stop future emails arriving. Our job is to deal with the content of the email which in this case would be financial issues.

As we chatted about previously, if someone is anxious about money, they could work on money. If someone is depressed in their relationship, they could work on their relationship issues and so on. Anxiety and depression are feedback, guiding you to work on your life. When you resolve your money problems and relationship needs, related emotions won't be there.

Now if you are consider taking medication to stop emotions, you are stopping the emails from arriving. **Your subconscious mind is now blocked from providing you with feedback**. You can't solve an emotion, but you can get to work on solving problems which will genuinely give relief and where you can be proud of yourself for personal growth.

Side-effects of any medication can be unpredictable. It is also unpredicted what will happen when you stop using medication. Anxiety and depression may come forth harder and stronger much like receiving 30-40 emails at once.

Consider, if your therapist's methods worked, why is it they administer medication to supplement that? Does the Therapist believe in your ability to transform outside of a medication/drug model? Do you believe this is possible? A plan to deal with negative self-talk, feelings of grief and loss, poor eating habits and relationship issues would be apt.

NOTE: If you are currently undergoing treatment, I am in no way suggesting cessation of medication. My suggestion is in truly looking after yourself before trekking down this path. I am of the belief that people progress through emotional difficulties. It's origin in working with thousands of people, watching them change the conditions of their life.

None I have ever worked with have changed their emotions, they changed the conditions of their life – that's what made the difference.

I was once on medication for anxiety, after 30 days I realised I hadn't felt a single emotion the whole time. I was existing, but not living so I stopped taking the pills and worked through anxiety and fatigue, my own way. I started on a path to deal with *being* a human being.

The medication model is designed to correct imbalance, but the medication also causes an imbalance of its own, which can't be predicted. Side effects can be very serious. Some medication prescribed for depression can have a side-effect of depression. Insomnia medication can have a side-effect of sleep problems. These are genuine side effects, no fabrication on my part.

In general, other side effects may include weight gain, loss/gain of appetite and a decrease in sex drive. Not eating well, gaining weight and a lowered sex drive would no doubt be an added source of depression!

Certainly there are positive experiences but many experience poor results and side-effects. It's often a best guess scenario in receiving appropriate medication. An anti-anxiety pill for a sleep problem or an anti-depressant pill for anxiety is authorised more often than you think.

The **empowerment model** assumes one has internal resources that correct imbalances. An effective holistic model addressing thoughts, emotions, body, relationships, food intake, exercise and other support structures. Personal power, before pill power!

Depression

Case Study Robert

How often do we allow time and space to really look after ourselves?

I was inspired by a client I worked with in 2015, named Robert. He had been working 60-70 hours per week for 10 years straight in corporate and charitable projects. He was overwhelmed by his life. What Robert did was take 4 months off from all his commitments. He said, "I have to get my life in order."

During this period he stopped work, got his finances up to date, began eating well, started exercising and was successful at quitting smoking. Robert stated that nothing was incomplete now and he would return to work on reduced hours.

In a decade of consulting with clients never had I witnessed a person dedicate that much time to looking after themselves. It was inspiring to witness. I believe he had taken that much time because he was out of balance for so long. You may not require several months to change your life. You could spend a week, or a weekend, tidying up things that most need your attention.

The purpose of depression is to alert you that your methods for dealing with life aren't currently working. There is nothing wrong with you. **Depression informs you that something within yourself and your environment are out of balance**.

You could write a list of all the messes that need tidying up in your life and show leadership in those areas. Start with one conversation or one room in the house. Create space so good things can enter your life again.

Identity: Who You Are

I want you to remember that addiction is not your identity. You are not your behaviour. Begin to separate *who you are,* from what you do. We chatted about identity and body image earlier on in the chapter on food. Let's examine further how identity can be so powerful.

Consider these two statements:

"I am an addict."

"I have a behaviour problem."

Many people are labelled an addict and given a treatment plan based on this identity diagnosis. If for a few seconds I picture myself as an addict, my thoughts actually drift toward addictive behaviours. The identity is where your beliefs and actions flow from.

On the other hand, if I were to picture myself as a person doing a *behaviour*, I can stop the behaviour. I can substitute it for something else that makes me feel good. I can deal with challenges that come up when I stop. I am not my behaviour, so I don't have to change me. I don't have to give up a part of me, to be a better me.

You could have been correctly labelled just about anything at some point in your life.

30 years ago, if a man committed murder, they would at present be labelled a murderer. It is a fact that it happened, but it would not be the whole truth about this person. What if over the next 30 years the then labelled murderer follows a philanthropic path, saving thousands of lives by dedicating their life to others.

Is this person a murderer? Humanitarian? Both? Neither?

An acquired identity sticks because of how you, or someone else feels about the behaviour that was done. The more proud or ashamed we feel, the more we believe that is *who we are*, which in my opinion would certainly warrant careful examination. Is a person forever to be labelled either saint or sinner?

Nelson Mandela once said, "I am not a saint, unless you think a saint is a sinner who keeps on trying." Is he implying there are many parts that make up who he is, not just a small portion of his behaviour?

He reconciled both sinner and saint in himself and was adamant not to be identified as either. For Nelson Mandela knew that the then prejudiced labelling was not to be a part of a future unified South Africa.

Identity: Who You Are

We find unity with parts of ourselves, by not identifying with them.

When a person holds the belief of the label that was slapped on them, they will find it nearly impossible to act from any other place, except from that label. It does not empower you to reach the potential you can. Go ahead now and set your old label down. It's not who you really are.

I bet you've tried to do something great before, but people took it the wrong way and you ended up being labelled something **nasty**. I bet you've even done something nasty, but it accidentally turned out great, so you were labelled **terrific.**

None of the things you've done have anything to do with who you are (identity). Can you see how identity is so open to interpretation? The learning here is that, not only is your behaviour not your identity, identity is also based on how someone feels about you.

So who are you now? You are not a label. You are not your addiction. You are not what someone thinks and feels about you. It is your decision who you would like to be. In fact, the identity you give yourself is the most important one there is.

It is really hard to change who you are as a person. Instead, realise that an acquired identity is not actually who you are. If you are not any identity, you can choose to be whoever you want to be in this moment. Your true identity is unlimited potential!

The prime minister or president of a country is labelled many different things. The way they function each day is to know that opinions are not the truth about them. To one part of the electorate, they may be seen as deceitful and to the other half a caring president of the people.

I have been strong and weak in my life. I have been mean and nice. I have been happy and sad. I have felt attractive and repulsive. I have been a sinner and a saint and these are all true for everyone. At some point in life we have to say, "My identity is not a one-sided judgement, about a tiny portion of behaviour, my worth is in the love I give today."

What others label you should not influence your identity and self-worth. You're not too different from the president, except you haven't decided whom it is that you are yet. Perhaps you have believed the labels that others have given you. If your current identity empowers you, keep it. If not, lay it on down to rest and try on a new one.

To determine if your identity empowers you, check in with the results you produce.

- You set goals you believe in and take action on them.

Identity: Who You Are

- You accept yourself, regardless of what others say.
- You set standards about how you are treated by people.
- You recognise positive and negative qualities in yourself and won't be defined by either.
- You take responsibility for results, over blaming others.
- You believe you are a valuable person.

Any belief about yourself that says you cannot do something, consider retiring it. Perhaps that belief protected you and kept you from trying, so you would not get hurt. The trouble with being protected is it also keeps you stuck. You can choose any behaviour you want to right now. You are not bound by a false identity any longer.

You are limitless potential.

You are a being capable of making contribution to others and living a full life, no matter where you are at right now. That's the truth. There are some things you wish you hadn't done, and parts of you, you wish were different, and you can also choose that is not who you are.

Your identity might be a hard one to deal with. Can you learn from it? Can you display better behaviours from today onwards? Can you be grateful for ways you already are magnificent? Can your experiences be used to impact people in a positive way?

Whatever you place in front of 'I am' is the most powerful statement you make to your world. The next time you are in front of your kids, boss, employees, husband or wife, make a new statement about who you are. Invent a new you to become, and act from that place.

Think of yourself as a radio station sending a message about who you are. People know you by what you broadcast to the world. What we unconsciously think of ourselves is written all over our face. There was a time when the story of my life was, 'unlucky with women.' When meeting women it was as if there was a big label on my head stating this and once they picked up on Jeremy is unlucky with women, it became a self-fulfilling prophecy.

I couldn't catch a break and for 10 years I couldn't meet the right woman. You start to believe the story and that makes you desperate. Not an attractive quality when trying to attract a mate! When engaging with women, I felt intimidated. We would start talking and I wouldn't know what to say next.

I would get flushed and to avoid embarrassment, pretend I had to leave, or stand by silently.

Over a period of time I started changing the story. I saw that many of the women I was intimidated by, I actually had no interest in. The irony was, I was nervous around women that weren't my type and was always comfortable around ones I truly liked. I created a new belief that, when I'm talking with the right woman at the right time, it just works.

Identity Opportunity: Who You Become

Perhaps people have come to know you as Peter the addict, Debbie the smoker, or Sharon always 10kg overweight. Because of Sharon's default identity, she can try multiple diets to lose weight and end up gaining it all back in an agonising cycle. What is the identity that could turn this around? Perhaps 'Sharon Never Gives Up,' or 'Super Fit Sharon.'

Identity does not have to be based on the one thing you feel worst about, it can be powerful, like who it is that you want to be. You can approach your world with a new energy, Pete the Triathlete, Debbie the Super Mum, Super Fit Sharon. Try one of these identities on for a while. Observe what you would do differently, if your identity was Super Fit Sharon (*or insert your new identity here*).

Likely you would be out exercising, encouraging others to join and eating better! Your body and mind will respond to new beliefs you carry about yourself.

Why not believe you are Super Fit Sharon, Debbie the Super Mum, or Pete the Triathlete, that's how all great people start, with belief in themselves that they will become that person. Act from your new identity every day.

You are no longer Pete TRYING not to be an addict. You are Pete looking after health and fitness to BECOME a triathlete.

Honesty alert: I decided to become a triathlete in 2013. I was running regularly and even took lessons from a former Olympian on how to swim properly. After 2 weeks of swimming my shoulder froze up badly. Combining this with a genuine dislike of cycling, I stopped triathlon training and switched to long distance running instead.

This was a better fit for me (refer to 'The Easy Way to Be Disciplined' chapter). Doing a thing you enjoy means you are far more likely to follow through with it. I chose something different, that worked for me.

It took several months of training along with smaller races in the build up to a half marathon. The day before the race my back seized up. I could barely walk or get up out of a chair without wincing. I never once thought of not turning up to the race. I told myself, "My back must be preparing me for the run." I believed it would be okay by the next morning.

I was invested in both identity and belief that somehow it would work out. My back was almost 100% free the next day and I finished the run. All of this and the day before I couldn't even bend over properly without pain. Some might say it was chance that healed it in time. I know better. **Belief** has made very unlikely things happen too many times.

Whilst dealing with chronic fatigue and quitting regular substance abuse, statements to myself were, "I am sore, I am angry, I am exhausted." I replaced these with new 'I am' statements, until I felt it in my body. I did this twice daily for 30 days.

You've tried on "I am an addict" or "I am useless" before. Try on these new beliefs below and feel them in body. Sit with each word and feel what actions you might take if you embodied these beliefs. Use these with your health, exercise or other life goals.

- I am strong.
- I am healthy.
- I am whole.
- I am complete.
- I am forgiven.
- I am compassionate.

- I am light.
- I am love.
- I am successful.
- I am a finisher.
- I am grateful.
- I am open to change.

A new identity is not created by *changing* identity. It is about realising who you really are. You are a being capable of choice. Beliefs place both opportunity and limits on yourself. Beliefs imposed by yourself or others are stories that you either accept or not. What identity and behaviours can you choose now?

Environment

We take on qualities of the 5 people we spend the most time with. When I think about the people in my life, I see there is a strong commonality with personal growth, business, healthy eating and nature. It is similar on my social media accounts. The people I interact with most, do many of the things I do.

Groups of family members, friends and workmates tend to create an unconscious agreement about what everyone in that group does. There is a spectrum of behaviour that everyone tends to abide by. If all members keep roughly similar levels of health, wealth and general acceptable behaviour, everyone stays content.

What happens if someone disturbs one of these unwritten agreements? What happens if one person decides to step out of line and increase their health and personal power? What if they decide to quit drinking or start running triathlons? The rest of the group will resist.

When you increase or decrease standards in life, beyond the 'normal identity' for your group, expect them to challenge you on that. The group may criticise and even ridicule you for a decision. This is the 'house rules.'

As you change behaviours, they will try to give you a new identity. You aren't like them anymore. Let's say you're working on getting fit, the group might label you 'gym junkie,' because they feel dis-identified with you. (We see yet again how quickly an identity is put together, sometimes constructed from a single new behaviour).

The solution here is not to completely stop seeing old friends, but to start making new ones. Seek people who are above the level you want to achieve and start spending time with them. The new friends you make will probably label you 'inspirational' or 'fitness machine.'

Don't listen to criticism from someone who is trying to bring you down. In fact, invite those friends to join in your new success. Rather than defending your position, invite them to examine theirs! Doing this keeps you in a position of strength and you may just motivate them to step up. Why would you invite them to join you? A few reasons:

- They form part of your new group and are not rejected.
- You achieve things with people you care about, not just on your own.

Environment

- It avoids you having to defend your decision, thus keeping you in a position of strength.
- You inspire and help others you care for.

Misery loves company... Yeah, but success loves company too!!

I consider whom to let into my world. Those who aren't adding to my health, wealth, business and fun are out. Not that these people are bad, there is just not a match between us right now.

In 2014 a friend sought more social togetherness. I would feel drained spending time with him and eventually ended this friendship, which wasn't an easy thing for me to do, as he was of gentle nature. 3 weeks later he'd moved out of his parent's house, purchased a motorcycle and lived with flatmates for the first time in years.

I mention this because you may feel a pang of guilt in moving on with your life. When you make the call of spending less time, they do find new people to support them. I stopped visits and he located others that were a better match for him. In fact, by letting go of those who don't match your life, you both have a real chance to flourish.

Over the last 7 years, I have tracked all of my relationships and friendships. I've had several people come and go and noticed that whenever one relationship ended, another one always arrived within an average of 3 days. The exact friend, family member, workmate or pet I needed was there for me.

I want you to think about a most significant person who has left your life. From that day to the present, make a list of every single person whom since have given you love, support, comfort and companionship. You may find it quite moving to see how many have been there for you.

When I was a starting out as a Hypnotherapist, I would spend time chatting with those at my level. As I advanced in work, I invested more of myself with clinic owners and successful professionals in my field. To rapidly advance in your health, wealth or quality of life, spend time in the company of **those with a higher level of success than you**.

Be okay being the least knowledgeable person in the room. Surround yourself by those you admire and some of their traits and ideas will rub off on you.

During fitness training days, I'd meet others doing the same. When I struggled being single, I had friends who were expert at meeting women. When I was building my business, 90% of friends were business owners. The people in your environment will change as you do and that's advantageous.

Don't get overly entangled in worrying about seeing less of one specific person. They may drift off for a while and reappear as both of you grow and develop. Notice that love is always there, perhaps it is in a form not yet recognised.

Addiction Buddy

When I look back at choices that display unhealthy behaviours, there always was an 'addiction buddy.' This is a person you tend to share your addiction with. There was cigarette buddy, marijuana buddy, ecstasy girlfriend, gambling friend and alcohol group.

Spending time with them means spending time with the addiction. Do you have someone in your life that is your addiction buddy? If you spend time with them, does it always lead to an addiction as such?

If you are serious about change, you are going to have to not socialise with people who trigger the addiction, unless you have other things in common. If all you ever do with someone is drink, gamble and use drugs, then that's probably all you'll ever do. Find activities together outside of what you would normally.

There are some pretty cool buddies out there you could choose from. You can change the identity of an existing friendship or deliberately seek one of these.

- Beach buddy
- Movie buddy
- Intimacy buddy
- Travel buddy
- Fitness buddy
- Business buddy
- Food buddy
- Sport buddy
- Fishing buddy
- Support buddy

People will either add or subtract value from your life experience. If the people around you over the last 5 years haven't changed, then life has probably stayed roughly the same. Diversity will not let you be less than who you can be. Nurture relationships with great people in your life.

Addictions as False Security

Addiction might feel like a friend that provides some form of security who has been part of your life for a long time and is stable amongst chaos.

The identity of being an addict may act as a form of security. It becomes something you hold on to. "I am an addict." It is safe. There is no risk of 'falling' when you are already at rock bottom. You know your daily routine, which brings with it a sense of security and comfort.

In the case of a cigarette smoker, an affair may ensue for 40 years or longer, having smoked 20 cigarettes a day which amounts to 290,000 cigarettes in their lifetime. Yes, in duration a person will have formed some connections with their addiction.

For some individuals the security of a compulsion or addiction is familiar and natural. It may feel like it's a part of them. There can be grief in giving up a long time seemingly reliable companion. Their grief may originate from losing their identity, the activity itself, or effects the addiction has afflicted upon them.

There exists a downside of security gained through compulsions and addictions, an addiction does not like to share! It doesn't like to share you. It will pull you away from family and relationships. You are more likely to be isolated or only around those who are similar.

At its worst, you will end up rejecting opportunities and those who want to be close to you. You will lie to family about where you have been and what you were doing. You will spend an extraordinary amount of energy in managing the addiction and excluding people around you.

Isolation allows you not to have to deal with people. After all, they are the ones trying to take away the security of your addiction. Compulsions and addictions could have you excluding people in the following ways.

- In maintaining it, you will spend large amounts of time away from people.
- You will deceive and lie to do it.
- You will hide money to fund it.
- You will avoid finding a life partner, so none can find your secret.
- You won't be present with people because you are thinking about sneaking away to do it.

Addictions as False Security

When you are addicted, you miss out on all that make life worth living. You think a 'security blanket' is there for you, but it is minimising your life. It stops you from deeply connecting and dealing with what's going on around you.

When it comes down to it in the end, lying in a hospital bed, shoes, gambling, cigarettes, or booze will not be there holding your hand. It will be people. Relationships are amazing and risky. They hurt and also are what will save you.

There are sources of real security that WILL be there for you. These are the sources of security that count.

- Your home.
- Your family.
- Your network.
- Your friendships.
- Employment.
- Your business.
- Your skills.
- Your education.

- Your intelligence.
- Your ability to make choices.
- The security of having money.
- The security of available information online.
- Security of spiritual understanding.
- Being present with your own breathing, water and food.

Possible realisations to garner from this chapter:

1) Start to see, that as a false sense of security develops along with your compulsion that it actually takes you away from other true securities. Addiction erodes security you currently may have.

2) If, at present you are missing a great number of securities listed here, could your life path include reclaiming these now? Building up these securities gives you a platform for an empowered life.

Addictions Compensate for Your Unfulfilled Voids

Case Study Debbie

Debbie, a lady I worked with on food control issues, realised her overeating was related to missing connection with her Mum. She believed that when she was younger, it was sweet food that was provided as a primary source of love by her mother. She duly noted, "Mum didn't really show me love in other ways."

For Debbie, food meant giving love. So if you're like Debbie, more food = more love. **The compulsion to eat more is attempting to fill a void of lacking something**. Food was the source that brought Debbie the most comfort and reminded her of love from her Mum. This is not something she chose consciously. This is however what was driving her overeating.

At home she cooked for her family every night. She gave love to her children through providing food, which is not a bad thing on its own. What Debbie was uncomfortable with, was the amount of food she and her children were eating. The type of food (refined sugar) also was concerning her. Weight gain, guilt and fatigue were telling symptoms that something was out of balance.

Food had become a primary source of love and reward in her family, as she had experienced with her Mum. Together, through our conversations we explored new ways that family could connect and feel rewarded with each other, that didn't include food at all.

We want to preserve love in the family and make sure food is not the only method they get it. They will continue sharing meals together. It will be a *part* of how they connect but will not be the only way.

If food is a primary source of love and you are missing love, you may find yourself over-consuming, to gain that feeling.

The new, working addictions model **WARP** recognises that you have needs and some of these are satisfied by corresponding behaviours. (Drinking, smoking, food cravings, sex addiction, gambling). You don't use these because they're bad, you do due to feeling like you're missing something without them.

Debbie felt she was missing love, food reminded her of special memories with her Mum. Compulsions and addictions provide you with something. At a deeper level ask, why do I do this? What positive intention do I have for keeping this in my life? What alternatives will satisfy that? When you get those answers, everything shifts.

Addictions as False Security

People aren't bad; behaviours aren't bad; they are trying to gain or avoid something in their life. Below is a list of things procured from a compulsion or addiction. This covers most major reasons for addictions. Use this as a guide for helping yourself and others.

Note that every reason listed is either a moving towards behaviour (trying to get something) or a moving away from behaviour (trying to avoid something). As human beings, we are always seeking to gain or avoid.

"Why do I do this?" "Why do I keep falling off the wagon?" "Why won't my husband/wife/son/daughter/friend just quit?" If you have ever asked one of these questions, the list of 50 reasons will provide insight.

People are getting their wants and needs met by their addiction. This is why they don't simply quit and why there is a relapse. A compulsion or addiction is serving a purpose and until the person finds a higher purpose or something to take care of their needs, one cannot expect a transformation.

List of 50 Reasons People Have Compulsions and Addictions

1. Feel pleasure
2. Treat/reward self
3. Energy boost
4. Feel comfort
5. The rush
6. Fit in with people
7. Connect with friends
8. Connect with partner
9. Connect with self
10. Lower inhibitions
11. Appreciate music
12. Appreciate art
13. Anticipation of act
14. Enjoy the ritual
15. Quick and easy
16. Increase arousal
17. Increase creativity
18. Increase sexual stamina
19. Increase sexual pleasure
20. Ease withdrawals
21. Feel special (Shopping)
22. Feel invincible (Cocaine)
23. Keep weight down
26. Avoid pain
27. Avoid issues
28. Stop anger
29. Stop boredom
30. Relieve stress
31. Have fun
32. Please others
33. Avoid thoughts
34. Feel in control
35. Lose control
36. Feel free
37. Function at work
38. Function at home
39. Get high
40. Bliss out
41. Feel normal
42. Feel ecstatic
43. Feel confident
44. Distract self
45. Get to sleep
46. Win money (Gambling)
47. Feel love (Ecstasy)
48. Drown sorrows

Addictions as False Security

(Drugs)
24. Have a break at work
(Cigarettes)
25. For spiritual insight
(Hallucinogens)

(Alcohol)
49. Create order
(OCD)
50. For a job
(Actors, Police)

Addictions Create What You Don't Want

It is valuable to gain perspective of the whole picture. Although addiction has benefits in the short term, it also causes the opposite of what you want in the long term. It's true that you receive pleasure from addiction but you also are creating, synchronously, an equal amount of pain.

Have you started to see reasons WHY people have compulsions and addictions? They are trying to get some of their wants and needs met, through their behaviour. It is also not really working. I consult with users taking ecstasy to get high and their life is in shambles. I work with smokers who still are very stressed and anxious. I work with drinkers who are mentally struggling to manage their life.

- The more you use speed to get high, the more drained of energy you become over time.
- The more you use marijuana to bliss out, the more paranoid and agitated you become.

- The more you use food for comfort, the more uncomfortable you become with your body (bloating, reflux, weight gain and other symptoms).

- The more you try to win money gambling, the more you lose over time.

- The more connection sought on social media, the more disconnected you become elsewhere.

- The more you drink alcohol to have an amazing night, the worse your hangover will be.

This is physics, expressed in psychology. Every action has an equal and opposite reaction. It is not possible to have a purely pleasurable experience in life. By all means do not take my word for it on this truth, go out and observe your life. Every high has an accompanying low. Addictions will not work.

My use of the ecstasy drug happened over a period of 3 years. I would go out and party to music all night and experience euphoria. Ecstasy provides some of the energy that speed does as well as feelings of love and instant connection with people.

Having sex while on ecstasy can be mind-blowing. There usually are deep feelings of love and connection – you know how to make all the right moves. A girlfriend and I had always been attracted to each other, but could no longer find that connection unless we were taking drugs. Over time, ecstasy wore away any natural attraction we had together.

The highs from a night out, bring lows over the following hours and days. Comedowns would often include insomnia, lethargy for days, sore muscles, a depressed mood, loss of connection and stomach cramps. There are always ups and downs. On balance, ecstasy presented me with experiences that had equal amounts of euphoria and pain.

Ecstasy caused feelings of love and connection. Ecstasy also caused a loss of love and connection in the long run.

Coffee and sugary drinks followed a similar pattern. The more I had, the more I needed to keep my energy up. Only when I gave it all away, did the body adjust and restore stable energy patterns. 7 years on and energy sustains over 80% every day. The more coffee or sugar you have, the more you think you need it!

No addiction is wholly negative or positive. Every addiction has equal benefits and drawbacks to doing it. Every high has a corresponding low. Every pleasure has a corresponding pain. Every stimulation has a corresponding depression.

Addictions Create What You Don't Want

Anything that is used as a stimulant, will create a short term depression. You will experience this as energy loss (physical), emotional imbalance (depression, worry, guilt) or mental imbalance (negative thoughts). Depression is a counter-balance to being overstimulated.

The purpose of depression may be to guide you away from overstimulation and fantasy (unrealistic) thinking.

You may relish the positive feeling of buying shoes, winning at gambling or using drugs for 3-4 days but a low will come. While buying your dream pair of shoes for the 16th time, you're not present to how meaningless these will be in a few days. At the time you're thinking how they perfectly pair with your outfit.

The pair of shoes, the gambling win, or the high from drugs will be meaningless in a very short space of time. The meaning you seek through the compulsion you have, is very short lived. You *crave* more because it is not satisfying you.

Note: There is nothing 'wrong' with behaviour of any sorts. The point here is seeing how deeply unsatisfying behaviours are in just a short space of time. Do you remember earlier when we spoke about false cravings? For example, hankering after new shoes is not for shoes, it is for what shoes do for you – perhaps used to feel good, elevate status amongst peers, or as a treat.

I believe it is important to look at humans being holistically. We can no longer say, "Stop doing that, it's bad." We need insight, understanding and creative solutions to satisfy what an urge is really about.

The more you use an unhealthy habit to attain a feeling, the MORE you cause its opposite. You are not meant to get attached to something damaging, which is why behaviours also cause the opposite of the desired effect.

There are reactions and counter-reactions (chemical and hormonal) making sure you live a balanced life. Over a period of 48 hours you will experience both equally.

We have glimpsed how an addiction works. There is always a positive intention and it always causes the opposite effect over time. It is a trap if you are chasing only positive feelings through addiction.

The Trap of Addiction: Chasing the Highs

Addictions Create What You Don't Want

The trap is belief that addiction will solve your problems. Including traps of additional gambling to recover losses, smoking cigarettes to recreate stress relief you once experienced, or taking ecstasy to get back sexual confidence you once revelled in.

Your behaviour is currently causing a problem, but you remain convinced of trying it yet again to recover results you have had before. This is 'chasing the highs.' Chasing things you've formerly experienced and it works only if you increase the dose. You are not designed to function like this.

Beware of chasing the highs – trying for what you had before.

The moment you realise you cannot function, is the time to stop. At this point a compulsion may cross over and become a dependence. Once there is dependency on a damaging substance, we are trapped. Addiction may be perceived as a familiar friend but it is the problem.

When I required ecstasy to have great sex, I knew then it was time to stop. I struggled in accessing connection which was easier before. If I used ecstasy to keep chasing the highs of sex, it would have taken me that much longer to undo the damage. Within is a natural ability to heal and experience pleasure in healthy ways.

There is supposed to be highs and lows – support for safety, and challenge for growth. **Depression and addiction arise when there is an expectation of highs without the lows.** We are addicted to a false reality, which real life does not match up to.

We wish life were different from how it is actually, chasing highs rather than finding satisfaction and being grateful with life as is. The thing you think you need, IS the thing that holds you back. I thought numerous things were needed to function properly. I see clearly now that every high I chased has come with a corresponding low.

Revealing What You Need

Case Study Nicole

In December 2017 I saw Nicole who had been using cigarettes to relieve stress and boredom. A single mum to 3 kids who ran a business from home for near on 20 years. She gave her "everything" to her kids and business.

She was stressed and smoked whenever she saw a gap longer than 5 minutes. I raised questions of whether she was the sort of person who moved from one task to the next without a pause or stop; or if cigarettes had become **the only way to relax and have time to herself**.

This rung true and she recognised why she had been smoking for so long. For every 5 minutes spare between her responsibilities, she smoked. Cigarettes had become the primary way for her to have a time out!

A great number of people I work with are disciplined and dedicated in parts of their life and an unhealthy habit provides a way to be free from all that responsibility. It is a way to have a little treat for themselves, release the pressure and not have to be in control.

The reason we do something, also shows us the way to leave it behind. She used cigarettes to get time to herself and affirmed that it had sorely been missed.

Nicole's interest peeked as she recognised just how bored and stressed she was, all the while smoking. It's not like cigarettes were working! Shocked they were adding to the stress (originally she thought it a reliever of stress). She avoided the kids, her issues and boredom overtook as she sat around smoking and not really living.

She exclaimed at the end of her session, "Smoking is stress!" Through our careful examination, she found several ways cigarettes were actually the cause of her stress. Although her intention for smoking had been relief, it reached the point where cigarettes had become a burden. They caused a lot more stress, than relief.

Nicole is working on **feeling better** and finding **time for herself** in ways she **enjoys** and are **healthy**. She **solves problems** as they come up rather than avoiding them. Why would she go back to cigarettes if they are costing her health, money, peace of mind and adding to her stress? She wouldn't. She didn't.

This is the sort of completion we will work together on for you. What you do has positives. The positives you seek, show you types of replacement behaviours to satisfy your needs.

Once you see alternatives that work and that the addiction causes what you actually don't want, you have transformed forever. You can't unlearn that truth, when it impacts you.

Not everyone is aware of why they do what they do. "I'm addicted" and "it's a habit" are surface level descriptions of what is going on for a person. A cigarette smoker wanting to quit might fear getting angry, worry about gaining weight and be unsure how to spend time with her husband who still smokes.

In this example, by continuing to smoke, cigarettes alleviate the fears associated with cessation. When she contemplates quitting smoking, fears will block her from following through for she has needs that must be taken care of. It is wise then to address **nicotine cravings**, **anger**, **relationship issues** and maintaining a **healthy weight** for this person.

It is often a stubborn or guilt ridden mind that stops people looking for genuine positives from their addiction. Having read the table of 50 benefits of addiction on page 133, you might still conclude that what you do is bad. It may have negative effects... however a question to consider is, if it all was bad, why do you still do it? Sit with this question and be open to what answers come up for you.

In asking these questions you are not condoning or allowing the behaviour to continue, you are discovering what you truly need in life. Without searching for the genuine positives you get from addiction, change will be unsustained.

- If you drink to forget problems, a pathway to solutions could include working on issues directly or finding healthy distractions.

- If you eat a lot of sugary food, you could be missing sweetness. Your path may include seeking sweetness through relationships, spirituality or material means.

- If you use cigarettes to keep calm and reduce stress, it may require getting your need of stress relief met in new ways and solving problems.

- If you over-use sex to feel connection, direct yourself in getting connected with your own physical body, spirituality or the world at large.

- If you use addiction as an attempt to escape life, is it time to escape your terrible job or partner? Travel or escape your current environment?

The reason we undertake something shows us our hidden needs. Let's say you have a regular habit of getting home and drinking a bottle of wine every night. You follow it like a ritual. It allows you to relax, takes your mind away from stress and you enjoy it. Is that close, wine drinkers?

The solution to changing this habit (as per your choice) is to **create a new ritual after work that allows you to fully relax, that you enjoy and takes your mind away from stress and problems.** When you decide to quit the habit of wine drinking, you have something to work with. This is FAR better than simply stating wine is bad.

Satisfy all key parts of wine drinking during times of consumption and suddenly you have options and control. What was once, "wine is bad and I can't stop" becomes; "wine has positives and I'm exploring all avenues to get what I want from healthy sources."

There is importance in knowing the hidden needs behind addiction. The reason you are engaged in something shows you the path to leave it behind. What do you get from your addiction? What else could you do to fully satisfy that?

The approach to be free from addictions includes physical and mental intervention.

Walker Addictions Removal Process (WARP)

In the pages ahead, you can work on your specific compulsion or addiction. I have used example addictions to demonstrate the **Walker Addiction Removal Process** in action.

There are 6 steps to the **WARP**, which can be completed in the blank tables.

1) Decide what compulsion/addiction you want to be free from. Write it down in the top section of the table.

2) Write down the benefits you get from your compulsion/addiction. As a whole an addiction is difficult to control. Broken into smaller parts it is manageable. You can use the 'List of 50 Reasons People Have Compulsions and Addictions' as a guide. I have included it again at the end of this chapter.

3) Write down 3-5 actions that would satisfy each of the benefits you wrote down. For example, if I'm working on the benefit of stress relief I would write: time spent in nature, exercise, solving the problem, massage and deep breathing techniques.

4) Reflect on whether the alternatives will genuinely satisfy the needs you have. They must be equal to or more satisfying than the addiction. For example, a gentleman I worked with on gambling is now educated in money systems and trades in a stock exchange. His needs of analysing variables, making money and sheer thrill are being fully satisfied by these alternative behaviours.

5) Write down all the negative effects of the compulsion/addiction. Include the things that are painful about it and the effects it has on you physically, emotionally, financially, socially and with family. Include answers that show the compulsion/addiction causes the opposite of your positive intention.

6) Ask yourself, "am I now completely free from this addiction?" If there is any doubt at all, return to step 2 and keep working. Once all of your needs and wants are satisfied, urges to return to the behaviour will be minimised.

Example WARP for smoking cigarettes

Compulsion/Addiction Smoking Cigarettes			
What **benefits** do you get from your compulsion/ addiction?	What **alternatives** can satisfy that benefit to the same or higher level?	Do the alternatives **fully satisfy the benefits** you listed?	In what ways does the compulsion/ addiction **negatively impact** you?
Relieves stress	Exercise. Spend time in nature. Swimming. Have fun.	Yes	Stress on my health. Stress of buying them. They stink.
Something to do	House work. Goal setting. Solve problems.	Yes	I'm bored. I waste so much time on them.
Helps me socialise	Maintain eye contact. Sincere listening. Find an interest in people.	Yes	Hard finding a place to smoke. Judgement by others. Have to leave people.
Enjoy it with a coffee	Enjoy food. Enjoy taste buds coming back. Conversations with people.	Yes	Can't even taste my coffee. I hate smoking. I feel guilty.
Avoid eating/ weight gain	Drink more water. Regular exercise. Eat consistently again.	Yes	Skipping meals makes my mind scattered. I feel out of balance. I'm so tired.

Smoking cigarettes gives you stress relief and other potential benefits, and it causes the opposite of what you are looking for. Stress about where you can smoke, when you can smoke, standing outside in the weather, lining up to buy them, anxious about how many you have left, feeling frustrated and guilty for smoking.

People experience guilt and worry about health, finances are under pressure, they dislike the odour and regard themselves as unsociable. They remark "I smoke to relieve stress"... However, you can clearly view it is also a cause of stress. Find alternatives for every reason you smoke and effective ways of reducing stress that are more advantageous to you.

Walker Addictions Removal Process (WARP)

Example WARP for eating chocolate

Compulsion/Addiction Chocolate			
What **benefits** do you get from your compulsion/ addiction?	What **alternatives** can satisfy that benefit to the same or higher level?	Do the alternatives **fully satisfy the benefits** you listed?	In what ways does the compulsion/ addiction **negatively impact** you?
Pleasure	Spend time in nature. Beauty treatment. Get a massage.	Yes	Sugar crash. Low energy. Bloating. Reflux.
Comfort	Hugs from family. A warm bath. Affection from pets.	Yes	Weight gain. Disrupts sleep. Uncomfortable in body.
The taste	Appreciate sweet, sour, bitter & salty foods. Enjoy seasonal fruits.	Yes	Tastes fake. Rots my teeth. I crave more & more, it's not satisfying me.
Reward/ Treat	Buy yourself presents. Do what you love. Time with people/ on own.	Yes	Weight gain. Foggy mind. Self- punishment.
Eating socially	Focus on people and connection. Enjoy other tasty foods.	Yes	Feel guilty. Worried about food habits. Financial cost.

Chocolate gives pleasure and other potential benefits, and it causes the opposite of what you are looking for. Discomfort in body, sugar crashes, low energy, disrupted sleep, weight gain, and foggy mind, unnatural taste, feeling guilty, temporary satisfaction, effects hypertension and diabetes.

You eat chocolate because it tastes great and it gives you pleasure. Too much and there are symptoms like guilt, low energy or diabetes, informing you of imbalance. Trust your body wisdom and adjust accordingly. It is not possible to have pleasure without pain. Your body lets you know when to make an adjustment.

Example WARP for using ecstasy

Compulsion/Addiction Ecstasy (drug)			
What **benefits** do you get from your compulsion/addiction?	What **alternatives** can satisfy that benefit to the same or higher level?	Do the alternatives **fully satisfy the benefits** you listed?	In what ways does the compulsion/addiction **negatively impact** you?
Feelings of euphoria	Spiritual work. Nature. Yoga Exercise. Meditation. Intimacy.	Yes	Energy crashes. Anxious. Depressed. Sore. Jittery. Headache.
Mind-blowing sex	Tantra. Sex and breath-work. Discover your sexual personality.	Yes	Can't 'get it up.' Can't 'finish.' More likely to get an STD. Painful.
Enjoy dancing	Dance at home. Social dancing. Dance at non-drug venues.	Yes	Sore muscles. Dehydrated. Fatigued afterwards.
Connection with people	Spend time with people you truly like. Build relationships. Self-acceptance.	Yes	Feeling disconnected. Connections via drugs are short lived.
Lowers inhibitions/ Increased confidence	Smile. Share your interests. Ask others about their interests.	Yes	Regretful. Feel out of control. Confidence is short lived.

Ecstasy leads to euphoric experiences and has various potential benefits, and it causes the opposite of what you are looking for. Mental and physical crashes, fatigue, feeling down, difficulty connecting with yourself and others, worried about getting caught by the police, more likely to make decisions you regret, higher risk of pregnancy, STDs and cheating on your partner.

There are dozens of ways to experience the highs of drugs from natural and healthy sources. If you do not currently know how to create ecstatic experiences outside of drugs and addiction, you are lacking a vital life skill.

Walker Addictions Removal Process (WARP)

Example WARP for problem gambling

Compulsion/Addiction Gambling			
What **benefits** do you get from your compulsion/ addiction?	What **alternatives** can satisfy that benefit to the same or higher level?	Do the alternatives **fully satisfy the benefits** you listed?	In what ways does the compulsion/ addiction **negatively impact** you?
Making money	Compound interest. Study money systems. Investing.	Yes	I lose more in the long run. Loss of trust. Loss of money.
The thrill	Foreplay and sex. Adventure sports. Service to others.	Yes	The thrill is very short lived. Going home empty handed.
To be sociable	Activities with people. Focus on people. Listen well.	Yes	I wasn't socialising. I was betting and avoiding life.
The uncertainty/ Randomness	Enjoy the uncertainty of nature, people and life itself.	Yes	A single bet is random, the house has a near certainty of winning.
To outsmart the system	Use your analytical skills at work. Invent something useful. Problem solving.	Yes	The system outsmarted me years ago. I'm still chasing losses that I can't recover.

Gambling provides exhilaration and occasional wins, and it also causes the opposite of what you are looking for. Loss of money, loss of trust from partner, loss of house or business, feeling out of control, feeling empty on the whole. Over time, gambling is not random, the system has outsmarted you years ago.

Winnings are geared to the house and away from you. Trying to reclaim the glory wins of the past is not a winning strategy. If you are always chasing your losses, you know what you are likely to receive – More losses. Finding purpose, connection and satisfaction all go a long way to making a healthy transition. Place a bet on yourself.

WARP Table

Compulsion/Addiction			
What **benefits** do you get from your compulsion/addiction?	What **alternatives** can satisfy that benefit to the same or higher level?	Do the alternatives **fully satisfy the benefits** you listed?	In what ways does the compulsion/addiction **negatively impact** you?
		Yes	
		Yes	
		Yes	
		Yes	
		Yes	

WARP Table

Compulsion/Addiction			
What **benefits** do you get from your compulsion/addiction?	What **alternatives** can satisfy that benefit to the same or higher level?	Do the alternatives **fully satisfy the benefits** you listed?	In what ways does the compulsion/addiction **negatively impact** you?
		Yes	
		Yes	
		Yes	
		Yes	
		Yes	

List of 50 Reasons People Have Compulsions and Addictions

Walker Addictions Removal Process (WARP)

1. Feel pleasure
2. Treat/reward self
3. Energy boost
4. Feel comfort
5. The rush
6. Fit in with people
7. Connect with friends
8. Connect with partner
9. Connect with self
10. Lower inhibitions
11. Appreciate music
12. Appreciate art
13. Anticipation of act
14. Enjoy the ritual
15. Quick and easy
16. Increase arousal
17. Increase creativity
18. Increase sexual stamina
19. Increase sexual pleasure
20. Ease withdrawals
21. Feel special (Shopping)
22. Feel invincible (Cocaine)
23. Keep weight down (Drugs)
24. Have a break at work (Cigarettes)
25. For spiritual insight (Hallucinogens)
26. Avoid pain
27. Avoid issues
28. Stop anger
29. Stop boredom
30. Relieve stress
31. Have fun
32. Please others
33. Avoid thoughts
34. Feel in control
35. Lose control
36. Feel free
37. Function at work
38. Function at home
39. Get high
40. Bliss out
41. Feel normal
42. Feel ecstatic
43. Feel confident
44. Distract self
45. Get to sleep
46. Win money (Gambling)
47. Feel love (Ecstasy)
48. Drown sorrows (Alcohol)
49. Create order (OCD)
50. For a job (Actors, Police)

Conclusion

What I attained from my former addictions is easily met now by exercise, games, intimacy, meditation, nature and my career. I no longer have an interest in the highs from compulsions and addictions, not because they aren't enjoyable but because these highs lack the freedom and richness I deserve.

There is no escaping the fact that addictions cause the opposite of what I really want to experience. This does not mean I will never have cravings again. I still do. The brain will search for previously had experiences when under pressure. Nevertheless when a yearning for marijuana arises around particular people, I know what to do. Here are the likely wants and needs to be satisfied.

- Appease the person offering it to me.
- Connect with people.
- Enjoy the ambience of nature.
- Enjoy sensations in my body.
- To 'be' in the moment.

These are some experiences I would enjoy, so I will satisfy those cravings. Not with the drug, but with life. Genuinely, I thank the person who offered it to me and focus on surrounding nature, or something beautiful. To experience joy from sensations in my body, I might go

Conclusion

for a swim or eat delicious food. I search for something enjoyable that is already in my vicinity.

In completing the **WARP (Walker Addiction Removal Process)** and following through, you can satisfy any craving.

I can write the top 5 things gotten from every drug I've taken and go get that from other experiences in life. Longing for drugs is a 'false craving.' It is all about having experiences that satisfy you. There might be a gradual progression of transformation as you discover more about *your* nature.

You are not limited by your environment. You are not limited by your identity and not by your subconscious mind. As we explored together, these contrivances can in fact work for you. This world is an amazing place. There is so much of potential outside of compulsions and addictions.

The more down and out you are, the more forward and upwards you can go. Your capacity for joy, growth and freedom is in direct proportion to the depth of pain you have experienced. When you're at rock bottom, you can only go up. It might not feel like it right now but your current breakdown is your breakthrough. What is hard will become easier as you get better.

Success after failure is the sweetest. Relief after grief provides the most peace. Joy after despair is the highest. Light after darkness is the most precious.

Don't replace an addiction with something else that is merely for pleasure or avoiding pain. Aim for healthy replacement behaviours that serve a purpose. Craving after intense pleasure and avoiding pain can be strong, but you are stronger. Do the **WARP** thoroughly and support yourself with new rituals.

Conclusion

The Power of Ritual

When rebuilding your life after a difficult addiction, you want to avoid stagnation at all costs. You want to sharpen your actions and thoughts, to cut through any chance of you having a slip up. A ritual is something that can focus your mind and strengthen your body.

I used to resist rituals as I felt like they were one more thing I'm being told to do! Rituals started out as an obligation, but became something I enjoy most of the time. Rituals were absolutely necessary on my journey of growth and I *filled my life* with what gave me the best chance of recovery.

The first and last hour of each day are your two biggest opportunities to create new rituals. The way you **start and end your day** will be in direct correlation with the way you live your whole life. Select 5 of the following to make up your morning ritual.

1) Walk/swim/yoga/gym before eating.
2) Drink warm water with lemon/drink hot tea.
3) Eat breakfast (within the first hour).
4) Meditation/being in nature/re-read this book.
5) Look at your goals and get started on them.

Upon waking is not the time to be checking emails, watching YouTube and consuming excessive caffeine. The above rituals are designed to put you on a winning path for the day. Do these every day for 60 days and you will change your life.

In the evening before sleep, slow things right down. A common house cat is a great role model for late in the day. They move slowly and purposefully. Cats are selfish and look after themselves. You can do the same. Select 5 of the following things to make up your evening ritual.

1) Read a book/listen to a podcast.
2) Have a shower/tidy your sleep space.
3) Do 20 minutes of meditation.
4) Write down 5 things you are grateful for.
5) Write your goals list for tomorrow.

Late at night is not the time to consume alcohol, attempt strenuous activity, or snack too close to sleep. I recommend a stop in over-stimulating your senses in the last hour before going to bed. Focus on being, rather than doing. Be like the cat, slowing down and looking after yourself.

An unfocused mind tends to slip back into depression and addictions. It is not enough to merely stop an addiction, you literally have to fill your life up with stuff that is beneficial for you. Choose rituals which support you and you love doing.

It is not possible to satisfy yourself with addiction. You crave more because it doesn't work.

Conclusion

There is no cutting back from addiction. If you're holding onto thinking you can be a casual user, you still have attachments to the behaviour.

I'd like to invite you to break through your addiction *before* you feel you are ready. It's one of the biggest secrets in life. No one is ever ready. There will be no time when it feels perfect to quit your addiction. You can do it now. Believe in yourself, more than you believe in the addiction.

Finish.

www.ingramcontent.com/pod-product-compliance
Lightning Source LLC
Chambersburg PA
CBHW071925290426
44110CB00013B/1482